breathless

PRAISE FOR *BREATHLESS*

"As an anesthesiologist, this book struck a deeply personal chord — both nostalgic and powerfully validating. It's an absolute must-read for surgeons, anesthesiologists, medical students, scrub nurses, techs, and anyone curious about the hidden world behind operating-room doors. The stories are extraordinary, the writing masterful, and the pacing utterly captivating. I couldn't put it down. This book didn't just meet my expectations — it blew them away."

Linda Bluestein, MD, Board-certified Anesthesiologist, Hypermobility Expert, and Host of *The Bendy Bodies Podcast*

"The most captivating medical dramas are what actually happens, not what's written for television. *Breathless* is more engaging than your favorite medical show. This book highlights the technical brilliance of surgery, and it's all brought to life with humanity, spontaneity, and suspense. You'll find yourself immersed in each case, as if you're right next to Dr. Lando, caring for these little humans, in a world where every second counts."

Alok Patel, MD, Clinical Assistant Professor, Stanford Medicine, Stanford Children's Health; ABC News Medical Contributor; and Podcast *Host, Patel It Like It Is*

"Dr. Tali Lando's *Breathless* is a delightful, thoughtful, and lyrical description of the challenges and triumphs of a Pediatric Otolaryngologist — a book that will be as intriguing to the public as it will be to her medical colleagues. It is exceptionally well written, and she takes her audience into her confidence as she explores various aspects of her career. Bravo to Dr. Lando for this accomplishment."

Samuel Barst, MD, Chief, Pediatric Anesthesia Department, Maria Fareri Children's Hospital of Westchester Medical Center

"This book is an amazing demonstration of writing for meaning-making and professional identity development, as well as an exploration of medical errors and triumphs, dedication to one's work and family, and the author's own illness journey with breast cancer. *Breathless* is an honest and compelling look at life as a pediatric otorhinolaryngologist, with reflections on the humanistic and surgical aspects of each case."

Rachel H. Kowalsky, MD, MPH, FACEP, FAAP, Associate Professor of Clinical Emergency Medicine and Clinical Pediatrics, Weill Cornell Medicine, NewYork-Presbyterian / Phyllis & David Komansky Children's Hospital; Winner of *The New England Journal of Medicine* Medical Fiction Contest

"If you're drawn to the intricate worlds and unforgettable characters of your favorite shows, then prepare to be captivated by *Breathless*. Dr. Tali Lando, a pediatric surgeon, invites you into the incredibly complex — yet surprisingly understandable — world of operating on children. This book, written with insightful detail and captivating storytelling, weaves together the specifics of Dr. Lando's practice with the deeply moving journeys of the children and families whose lives she has touched ... and who have touched her as well. Her stories are so compelling they deserve to be a wonderful television series in the making — *Breathless* delivers an experience you won't want to miss."

Kristin Bernstein, Television and Film Producer, *A Beautiful Mind, Only Murders in the Building*, and *The Sopranos*

"*Breathless* by Dr. Tali Lando is a powerful, deeply human account that reminds doctors why we went into medicine in the first place. As a pediatric ENT surgeon, Dr. Lando takes us behind the sterile doors and into the soul of the hospital — where lives are saved, sacrifices are made, and heroism is often quiet but relentless. From the sleepless nights to the red tape that threatens to break us, from the fierce dedication to the unshakable camaraderie of medical teams, this book captures the raw reality of medicine. It's a tribute to every physician who has ever held a life in their hands and an homage to the moments that remind us why we do what we do."

Sue Varma, MD, Board-certified Psychiatrist, Clinical Assistant Professor at NYU Langone Health, First-ever Post-9/11 Medical Director of the World Trade Center Mental Health Program, and Author of *Practical Optimism: The Art, Science, and Practice of Exceptional Well-Being*

"*Breathless* is a compelling memoir that pulls back the curtain on 'physician life,' welcoming readers into the realities of what many busy doctors face — navigating the competing demands of a high-stakes medical career, marriage, parenthood, and more. Dr. Lando writes with the authority and expertise of a seasoned surgeon and the vulnerability and heart of someone who inevitably sees her own daughters in the eyes of her pediatric patients as they invariably live and die, struggle and thrive. In the pages of is inspiring book, Dr. Lando captures the heartbreak and triumph of medicine, the messiness of family life, and the grit it takes to keep showing up. Her voice is candid, warm, and wise. Her resilience and commitment to both her patients and her family make for a heartwarming read. This book left me breathless — not only for the lives saved, but for the humanity in every page."

Lizbeth Meredith, Professional Speaker, Host of the *Persistence U Podcast*, and Author of *Pieces of Me: Rescuing My Kidnapped Daughters* (Now a Lifetime TV Movie)

"Tali Lando's *Breathless* is a testament to the precision, resilience, and compassion that define the very best of medicine. Through expert insight, detailed case studies, and powerful narrative, it brings to life the challenges and triumphs of caring for our most vulnerable patients. With her uniquely human voice, you feel like you're standing beside her as she recounts some of the most foundational moments of a fierce career. For young surgeons, it offers a source of profound inspiration — a reminder of why we choose this path and the lives we can change through dedication and skill. *Breathless* is a must-read for anyone entering the world of medicine or seeking purpose in their surgical journey."

Chris Park, MD, Otolaryngology - Head & Neck Surgery, PGY5, University of Indiana

"*Breathless* by Dr. Tali Lando is not just a collection of riveting medical stories—it's a rare window into the psychology of teamwork under unimaginable pressure. With honesty, clarity, and an unmistakable authenticity, Dr. Lando takes readers inside the operating room, where every decision is high-stakes, and every conversation matters. Her vivid storytelling lays bare not only the trauma, guilt, and exhaustion of a surgeon's life, but also the resilience, trust, and profound humanity that hold medical teams together. This book is as much about *people* as it is about medicine: the colleagues and mentors who provide strength in moments of despair, the nurses who hold it all together, and the leaders who cultivate trust and vulnerability. Each story reveals how effective communication, emotional intelligence, and deep respect for one another transform a group of individuals into a life-saving team. *Breathless* is a tribute to the courage and devotion of healthcare professionals—and an unforgettable lesson in the power of teamwork."

Michelle Brody, PhD, Clinical Psychologist and Executive Coach, Author of *Own Your Armor, Revolutionary Change for Workplace Culture* and *Stop the Fight! An Illustrated Guide for Couples*

"*Breathless* is a riveting and unforgettable read. Dr. Tali Lando captures the heart-stopping suspense of the operating room with the warmth and humor of a wife, mother, daughter, and friend. As someone who once led communications at a medical sciences university, I was especially moved by her fierce devotion to the residents she mentors and the tenderness she shows to her patients' families. She embodies the best of medicine — brilliant surgeon, compassionate teacher, humble colleague — and she also happens to be the most gifted physician-writer I've ever encountered. In her hands, the drama of high-stakes medical intervention and the everyday rhythms of family life coexist on the same page, equally compelling and deeply human. This book left me both breathless and grateful for the dedication of doctors like her."

Kate Colbert, Author, Marketer, Healthcare and Higher Education Consultant, Former Director of Communications at Rosalind Franklin University of Medicine and Science

"Dr. Tali Lando's *Breathless* is riveting and profound. A pediatric airway surgeon, Lando invites us into the high-stakes world of saving tiny lives, delivering her stories with a matter-of-fact clarity that feels like *Grey's Anatomy* meets *Law & Order*. The result is a book that blends the emotional intensity of medical drama with the sharp precision of investigative storytelling. Each chapter introduces readers to infants and children who became little heroes on the operating table, their stories narrated with meticulous medical expertise and deep compassion. The cases are gripping, the stakes life-and-death, yet Lando's writing makes complex surgical challenges accessible to everyone without ever losing the weight of the moment. *Breathless* quite literally leaves you breathless and on the edge of your seat as you follow these journeys from the brink of despair to miraculous recoveries. It is equal parts educational, heart-wrenching, and inspiring — a testament to both the resilience of children and the skill of the surgeons who fight for them. This is a must-read for anyone fascinated by medicine, storytelling, or the human spirit."

Jenna Michael, Author of *Let's Choose Less: A Young Family's Guide to Simply Living* and Founder of *Your Purposeful Parenting*

"*Breathless* is one of those rare books that takes hold of you from the very first page and doesn't let go. Dr. Tali Lando, a highly skilled pediatric airway surgeon and exquisite storyteller, takes us into the operating room, where the stakes are at their highest, giving readers a rare front-row seat to some of the most complicated and delicate surgeries, fighting for the lives of children — even infants. A mother herself, Dr. Lando champions her patients with unrelenting compassion, revealing to readers the quiet courage of medical teams and the emotional depth of a surgeon who shows up for others when they need her most. Written with heart, humility, and humor, *Breathless* serves as a powerful demonstration of what it means to sacrifice for others and to keep going, against all odds. Buckle up for an enthralling, inspiring, and mesmerizing book about what happens when a surgeon and her team perform the extraordinary to save and improve lives."

Emily Florence, Award-winning Writer, PR, and Digital Marketing Consultant, and Author of *Even Better: Easier Ways to a Happier Life*, recognized as "The Feel-Good Book of 2024" by Yahoo Finance

breathless

SURGICAL TALES FROM THE BRINK

(and back)

TALI LANDO, M.D.

PEDIATRIC AIRWAY SURGEON

Breathless: Surgical Tales from the Brink (and Back)

Published by Silver Linings Media, an imprint of Silver Tree Publishing.
Silver Tree Publishing is a division of Silver Tree Communications, LLC (Kenosha, WI).

Editing by:
Kate Colbert

Cover design and typesetting by:
George Stevens

Medical illustrations by:
Juliette Aronoff

First edition, August, 2025
Paperback ISBN: 978-1-948238-53-3
Hardback ISBN: 978-1-948238-54-0
Library of Congress Control Number: 2025914999

Created in the United States of America

DEDICATION

My father, Dr. David Lando (PhD), was the only person who relished every nitty-gritty detail of my operative cases. Every day, I dialed him immediately upon my exit from the hospital, the moment the automatic glass exit doors slid open and the blast of cold or hot air hit my face. He always listened intently without interjection or need for reciprocation. His interruptions were so infrequent that I often needed to ask:

"Aba [father in Hebrew], are you still there?"

"Yes, Tali, go on. I am here. I'm just fascinated."

With his untimely death in 2015 from a brain tumor, I forever lost that valuable retelling and processing opportunity — which I not only cherished but also clearly needed. My decision to write this book reflects that tremendous personal loss. Beyond that is a broader purpose. Embedded in these carefully selected cases are valuable life lessons. This book is a peek behind the curtain. Each story depicts a particular set of real life-altering events that forever impacted my patients and their families. But, as you will see, the aftermath and reverberations of our decisions, our failures, and our successes profoundly affects us surgeons too.

TABLE OF CONTENTS

FOREWORD

By Dr. Mike Rutter

MEDICINE — ESPECIALLY medicine that involves surgery — is fascinating, frightening, and can involve bewildering complexity, especially to the lay public. Consenting to a surgery involves, at least temporarily, giving up the autonomy of your own body to someone you barely know or may have only recently met — someone with scalpels and instruments and a great deal of scientific knowledge. But here's the funny thing about medicine — it's so much more than science; it is a nuanced interaction between science and *art*. And, when push comes to shove, it's also about instinct and intuition. A great surgeon balances it all, applying their well-honed skills, trusting their gut, seeking creative solutions, and pouring every ounce of their energy into the one single goal: good surgical outcomes for their patient.

Even the most gifted surgeons acknowledge that outcomes don't always relate to skill alone. While surgeons need to know a lot, it's just as critical for us to know what we *don't* know, to acknowledge our limitations, to be able to swallow our pride, and to know when to ask for help. There are so many things that may influence the outcomes of an operation, including things as diverse as the surgeon, the patient (including their genetics, race, and social status), and — slightly disturbingly — sheer blind luck. Through it all, patients and their families report that, in addition to valuing a surgeon with great skill and humility, having a *guide* who can speak with a clear voice — with empathy and honesty — is something to be treasured.

I have known Tali Lando for more than a decade. We are both pediatric otolaryngologists (kid's ENT docs). When we initially met, she had just written a book — *Hell and Back: Wife and Mother, Doctor and Patient, Dragon Slayer* — about her journey of survival following her breast cancer diagnosis. It was beautifully written, encompassing pain, passion, and family, in a message of hope defeating adversity. And while we initially connected professionally (Tali has some truly challenging patients, as this book will serve to illustrate), it was her humor and compassion that made us friends. Tali is a truly talented surgeon; she is also (and fundamentally) a wonderful human being. It is my personal experience that if you let even a little of her into your life, the experience of knowing her will expand your existence. Tali has the rare talent of knowing how to simplify the multifaceted components that comprise modern medicine. And this she somehow manages — delivering outstanding care and remaining committed to the demands of her patients — while also juggling the daily needs of her family. She makes it work but is open about the imperfections.

Many years back, I flew into New York from Ohio to speak at a Pediatric Airway Symposium. Tali was one of the hosts of the course. While I was speaking, she realized this was her chance to have me directly evaluate the airway of one of her challenging post-operative airway reconstruction patients. She refused to squander this rare opportunity. She snuck out of the room and called the care facility where the patient resided. She convinced the head critical-care physician to arrange for the patient to be urgently transported to the children's hospital that same afternoon. She begged the operating room head nurse and chairman of anesthesiology to open an operating room. Lastly, she reached the hospital administrator (who was out of town) and the physician in charge of granting emergency operative privileges.

She started each of these conversations with, "Do you want to move a mountain today for the sake of a patient?" She convinced all these people to fast-track approval for something that typically takes weeks to months. When she had all the signatures in place, she snuck back into the auditorium and waited for me to finish my talk. Then, she updated me with her plan: "Would you be willing to finish the conference and come into the OR with me if I have everything ready to go? It's too hard for the family to travel to Cincinnati to see you. I want your in-person opinion to achieve the best outcome for him. Please?"

It was impossible to say no. I think the term is "a Force of Nature."

"Just one more *little* thing," she added.

"I just need the chairman of your department to immediately send a letter to the chairman of my department vouching for you … and a copy of your medical malpractice coverage."

I mean you have to laugh (after the appropriate eye roll!). But the thing is, Tali made it happen. Straight from the hospital's auditorium, I followed her toward the lockers where she provided me with a pair of scrubs. Soon after, I trailed her down the OR hallway into the room where this child was already prepped with the airway equipment carefully pre-arranged.

This is who Tali is. This is why I answer her texts and calls — which typically begin with, "Mike, it's Tali. Have you got a minute? I have a little girl here who ..." For Tali, it's always about the kids.

Breathless is the kind of book that most physicians aspire to write but never find time to tackle. It is profoundly vulnerable and appropriately detailed from a medical perspective. It invites readers into harrowing and hopeful cases, where the stakes are high and the outcomes unsure. This book is for us all — a book about the inexact science of medicine. It's for those who aspire to go into medicine as a career and it's for patients (and families) who have survived agonizing medical ordeals. It's a book for surgeons as well as those who work with surgeons and understand the culture of the operating room, the aftermath of difficult cases, and the toll that it takes when you wake up every morning, devoted to saving and improving lives.

No matter who you are or where you are, this book has something for you ... something special, something surprising, something inspiring, and something that you will never forget.

Mike Rutter, FRACS, MD

Pediatric ENT Surgeon, and Director of the Aerodigestive and Esophageal Center,
Cincinnati Children's Hospital Medical Center

PROLOGUE

I AM AN adrenaline junkie. But not the kind who jumps out of airplanes, gets airlifted onto snow-capped mountains, or straps on a bungee cord and steps off a bridge. I am the kind whose blood-pumping, heart-dropping moments start with a call about a child in severe respiratory distress and end in the operating room, hopefully with the successful intubation of an impossibly narrow airway.

I am an adrenaline junkie who is petrified to break even my littlest pinkie. But I am not afraid of confronting the narrow pass between life and death. The only thing I really fear — the thought that jolts me awake from a dead sleep in a cold sweat — is ... failure.

I am a pediatric "ear, nose, and throat" (ENT) surgeon, most officially known by its Latin term as an oto-rhino-laryngologist. Sometimes, I feel more like a psychologist, allaying parent fears about surgery and anesthesia. Other times, I function as a marriage counselor, attempting to resolve parents' squabbles and profound discord in the interest of the child. Often, I feel like a sleuth, trying to solve the mysteries of an enigmatic clinical case that unnerves me. Mostly, I thrive on being a combination of these things — a patient problem-solver. Lastly, I pray that in my very best days, I am a well-trained healer.

Doctor, Patient, Author, Scuba Diver

Ten years ago, I was a patient. I was in the fight of my life against advanced-stage breast cancer. When I first read my pathology report with that big invasive tumor and those myriad nodal metastases, I was sure I would lose. So much studying, years of training, sweat, tears, and debt. So many missed family events, birthday parties, ruined relationships, and lost friendships. So much sacrifice …

Poof, just gone.

In my mind, I called my cancer "The Beast." With my squad of surgeons, oncologists, and radiation therapists, I manifested as "The Dragon Slayer."

I even wrote a book about it, entitled *Hell and Back: Doctor, Patient, Dragon Slayer.* To produce that first memoir took an amount of emotional and mental effort that I likened to birthing a fourth child, something I had always wanted but which cancer stole from me. During that grueling treatment year, in the doldrums of nausea and weakness from chemo-haze, I needed a clear purpose. I needed a reason to drag myself out of bed, get dressed and leave the house. If I was not a practicing physician (at least, temporarily), who was I?

During that grueling treatment year, in the doldrums of nausea and weakness from chemo-haze, I needed a clear purpose. I needed a reason to drag myself out of bed, get dressed and leave the house.

Once, as a girl, teen, and young adult, I fancied myself as a writer. I was a prolific producer of poems and short stories, all carefully preserved to this day by my doting mother, Susan, in organized and dated folders. Along the way, I got the "doctor bug." I stopped writing anything but dry journal articles. I directed all my energy into the attainment of my medical license and the completion of my residency and fellowship. This pursuit consumed the remainder of my college years, my 20s, and my early 30s.

When I was blindsided by breast cancer at age 36, I finally returned to my dormant passion for writing. With every gut-wrenching experience, I typed and typed. With every moment of levity, I tapped and clicked. Writing became my salve. I poured my soul into those pages. Every raw truth or humorous experience materialized into neatly consumable anecdotes. My ultimate goal was solidified: to channel both my pain and my triumph into a medicinal guidebook for others. Through my journey as a patient, I could be a doctor … still, somehow, against all odds.

What ultimately emerged was a compilation of my deep personal tapestry from diagnosis to the aftermath, the rejoining of life, the relaunch of my career, and my gradual transformation back to a recognizable self. When the manuscript was done and after countless rounds of editing, tightening, and perfecting, I submitted my "masterpiece" online. In one of the *many* rejection letters I received from the big and small publishing houses, a kind editor wrote, "Really loved the writing and your voice, but the subject matter is just *too* overdone. I'd be interested in a book about your life as a female surgeon who also scuba-dives. Feel free to get back to me when you write about that … good luck with your fight."

That message stuck with me through the battle and even when I re-entered the workforce. The idea was still nagging at me long after I, once again, became swallowed whole by the resumed responsibilities of wife, mother, and doctor. I stored that criticism/ complement in the recesses of my mind, always hoping that I'd live long enough to retrieve it. *One day, maybe, there will be another book*, I thought.

This time, I would tell my tale from a position of well-being rather than uncertainty — of strength rather than vulnerability.

So, here I am, just over a decade later (Thank G-d)[1], ostensibly cancer-free. Still standing.

And here are my stories, culled from the thousands of commonplace medical cases down to the unbelievable and fascinating few. These patient encounters are ones that really stuck with me, a completely de-identified amalgam of tales I found myself repeating so many times to my trainees and to my friends. Each one has a unique evolution, a lesson to learn, and/or a pearl of wisdom that added to my experiential necklace. Each one consumed my thoughts long after the case was complete or the medical mystery was deciphered.

Some of the circumstances of these patients' conditions are so improbable that they may seem unbelievable. But although all specific details — including names, gender, age, ethnicity, and sometimes even exact diagnosis — have been thoroughly changed to conceal identity (and comply with HIPAA, the Health Insurance Portability and Accountability Act), the core elements are all true.

I know because I was there.

So, settle in and buckle up, because their stories will leave you … breathless.

---

1. Writing "G-d" instead of spelling it out is a Jewish custom as a sign of respect.

G-d formed the Human from the soil's humus, blowing into his nostrils the breath of life: the Human became a living being.

GENESIS 2:7

G-d said, "My breath shall not abide in humankind forever, since it too is flesh."

GENESIS 6:3

BACKGROUND

THE STORIES THAT make up the 19 chapters of this book take place in a Level I Trauma Center in an academic regional referral center, where we care for patients from a very large catchment area of approximately 30 million people. The medical center has its own free-standing children's hospital. Because it is one of the few children's hospitals in the state, we get children flown in or brought in by ambulance from all over the region. The neonatal intensive care unit (NICU) admits more than 900 critically ill infants a year. Our pediatric intensive care unit (PICU) sees approximately 1,200 patients a year with all sorts of illnesses. Many of these patients require ENT consultation. The patients we serve come from extremely diverse backgrounds, ranging from the very wealthiest to the most financially destitute. As a result, the stuff we encounter can range from the ordinary to the most extraordinary medical "zebras."

The Operating Room

The operating room (OR) is a place of rituals. We cling to those rituals like a baby koala clings to its mother's belly. We crave this security because we all know the truth: that there are forces beyond our control, that despite decades of training and constant repetition and the precision of fine muscle memory, that there is an element of serendipity that governs our outcomes. We will do anything it takes to ward off bad surgical juju. We will don the same old ratty scrub cap from medical school under our new disposable Smurf-blue bouffants. A decade into our careers, we will wear the same tattered purple Dansko clogs that our mom bought for us on the first day of surgery internship despite the many bleach stains incurred while wiping off caked-on blood. As for me (an observant Jew), I'll knock on any piece of wood I can find (even though all the OR surfaces are metal) if it'll bring Lady Luck to my side that day.

We also prepare. We think about the difficult cases. We read up on them, even if we've performed them countless times. We lie in bed at night, playing various scenarios in our minds. We move the pieces of potential outcomes on the ceiling like a chess player in *The Queen's Gambit*. Although preparation is essential, no matter what advanced thought we give to our patients, things change. Unexpected twists and turns will present themselves and there will always be decisions to be made on game day. People always think that the most important part of being a surgeon is having "good hands." But listen closely because I will tell you a valuable secret: the hands can only do what the brain tells them to.

People always think that the most important part of being a surgeon is having "good hands." But listen closely because I will tell you a valuable secret: the hands can only do what the brain tells them to.

The Surgical Time-Out: A Brief History

The Surgical Safety Checklist (and its many elements) is affixed prominently on the wall of every operating room in our hospital, in one form or another. It is a written manifesto of the safety initiatives modeled on a checklist developed by the aerospace manufacturing juggernaut, Boeing, in the 1930s. The concept was that pre-flight checklists were shown to dramatically reduce airplane crash rates. This easily translated to the operating room and was proven to improve patient outcomes in positive ways.

The surgical time-out was introduced in 2003 primarily to prevent "wrong side," "wrong procedure," and "wrong patient" errors. There is a set of scripted questions that gets read aloud in addition to patient and procedure identification. The time-out is also used to introduce the patient to the operating-room team, and to provide an overview of their diagnosis and our intended treatment. The surgical time-out is supposed to be a sacred time of pause, in which all team members — anesthesia, nurses, scrub techs, and the surgeon(s) — communicate about the operative plan and its potential nuances. For example, in the field of otolaryngology, there is often a heightened fire risk. We often use electrocautery in proximity to oxygen and fuel sources. Accordingly, we use the time-out to alert the anesthesia team to lower the oxygen concentration to a non-combustible level during key moments of the case.

The time-out can also be used as a friendly primer to the day. "Good morning, I am Tali Lando, surgeon." The highly skilled, widely published, stunning dark-skinned bedazzled woman at the head of the bed with long curated eyelashes and perfect makeup (damn her) is Dr. Irim Salik, anesthesiologist. Franny, our loving

Italian long-time devoted ENT nurse, raises a hand by the computer. Christina, our feisty scrub-tech, nods from the instrument stand.

Most of the time, we all know each other really well already. I mean, we don't just know each other's names — we know all the details of our lives, recent tiffs with spouses, new romances, which of our kids is struggling with math, whose teenager is involved in a love triangle, stuff like that.

Christina is a petite white woman with thick black glasses who has lost more than 100 pounds in the past five years. She's also a whip smart, adopted ex-preemie born to a drug-addicted mother of distant Iraqi descent. She has two children. Her son, who almost played professional baseball, is now in trade school learning HVAC. Her daughter is in competitive cheerleading and just got into her first-choice college, aspiring to be a doctor.

Notably, Christina is also an OR sage — a wise woman, solver of problems, big and small.

"Where is the metal nut for the tonsillectomy suspension arm that adjusts the height of the lever?"

"How should I react when my daughter won't let me hug her anymore?"

"Where did I leave my hospital ID?" (Hint: it's always in the bathroom stall on the shelf above the toilet-paper roll.)

She also orders Crumbl Cookies to the hospital lobby when we've had a tough, long day or when we know it's shaping up to be one. My favorite flavor is key lime pie.

So, as you see, this required introduction is typically just a formality.

Much to my chagrin, every once in a while, a floating nurse (who I don't know) is surreptitiously inserted into our exclusive circle. This start-of-case introduction can then serve to break the ice. More importantly, it reminds me of their name. Otherwise, I'll spend the whole day saying, "Hey you, pass the scalpel."

The Debrief

The surgical debrief is a newer and less-accepted part of the operating-room culture. It occurs at the end of the case. It is supposed to be initiated by the surgeon but the discussion is open to all staff members to summarize what, if anything, we could have done better. The intention, again, is to improve patient safety, but it can also be used as a tool to enhance team communication.

For this book, I will use my own version of "the debrief" as a mechanism of highlighting the "take-away" that I teach my surgical residents and the ways in which each of these cases were remarkably impactful. This is how we grow from our experiences (both good and bad), how we adjust, and how we try to improve. It's one of the most valuable elements I have learned in my career so far. And, no matter who you are and what you do, medical or otherwise, you can learn from this too.

> This is how we grow from our experiences (both good and bad), how we adjust, and how we try to improve.

Surgery can be the most demanding and devastating profession. It can also be the most profoundly fulfilling. Taking care of other humans is a labyrinthine affair. The level of responsibility is almost unfathomable. The factors determining success are often untamable. It is not for the faint of heart.

The insights in the forthcoming chapters are gleaned from thousands of individual days, years, and over a decade and a half of high-volume patient care. They are the life lessons I have acquired through the blood, sweat, and tears of personal experience, triumph, and loss.

Accept this soul-searching literary offering for what it is. I do not have all the answers. No one does. But one thing I can say without hesitation is that I have definitely asked the hard questions.

At Home (The Spillover)

The spillover is not a technical term, and it is not an accepted part of the surgical ritual. Rather, it is the personal and emotional tax that these events levy on the surgeon. This is not at all an attempt to engender sympathy. I love my job, and I have no regrets, no matter what the cost has been. This is the life I signed up for, eyes wide open, and I am grateful for it. Still, it does take a very real toll. In this book, I will provide a window into the reality of the life of a surgeon. No matter what, operating on kids and being on call for bleeding and airway emergencies blurs the line between work and home life to an extreme degree. It also creates an unnatural hierarchy in which our obligation to our family — and to our children's needs and wants — is often superseded by our responsibility to others. This is something that my children have grappled with and, at times, resented, though they may not readily admit it. My stress, my mood, and my exhaustion at the end of the most grueling days often leave only crumbs for them and for my husband. I try to rally at night whenever possible — really, I do. So often, I crash hard and fail. I don't have some magical answer to the balance of it all, though I sure as hell wish I did. Many brave women and men before me have attempted to resolve this dilemma through some form of super compartmentalization. Maybe they have been successful, maybe not.

> Operating on kids and being on call for bleeding and airway emergencies blurs the line between work and home life to an extreme degree.

To them, I can only say honestly, I would too if I could. I do my best, but the reverberations of these intensive patient experiences echo loudly in my home life. Ask anyone with a job like mine.

MY COMRADES IN ARMS

SPEAKING OF PEOPLE with jobs like mine, I'd like to say a few words about my colleagues before we jump into the first patient case. In these specific medical battles, I am never the only soldier in the fight, keeping our patients alive and safe. In addition to my cherished otolaryngology compatriots, my colleagues in pediatric anesthesia are right there beside me, deep in the fray. Though we may occasionally squabble, become irritated over day-to-day incidents like delays or cancellations (usually when a child or their parent violates the "no eating before anesthesia" — "nil per os" or NPO — restriction), we really respect and value one another.

In our hospital, the pediatric anesthesia office is a small windowless room. Nevertheless, all the pediatric specialty surgeons hang out in this cramped space. Firstly, we do this because they have an espresso machine and often have food and snacks. They celebrate each other's birthdays with cake, and there's no "nothing by mouth" rule for the surgeons. More essentially, we cohabitate because our existences are so inextricably intertwined. Also, it happens we have no designated offices of our own (no lie). On any given day, we squish in there, even if it means sitting on the computer desks or drinking our coffee propped up against the dingy walls. It's not a glorious setting by any stretch, but still it's the nerve center of our daily social interactions.

It's typically early on a Monday morning when Dr. Sam Barst walks in, shooing me out of my seat, which is fair given the fact that I am actually sitting at his desk. Sam is the chief of the pediatric anesthesia department, a sharp double-boarded bespeckled classic father figure with an endless supply of cheesy (and only occasionally dirty) jokes. He guides his department by benevolent example, never flaunting his authority but setting a high standard of work ethic that he expects to be met. He is exactly my ideal leader. When my own father was dying, I sought refuge in his signature "life talks," basking in the familiar glow of brilliant introspection with a dash of corny Jewish humor.

That morning, I'm still rubbing my eyes and downing my first round of liquid caffeine when Irim bursts in — all glamour in her three-inch heels, flawlessly styled outfit, and runway-finished hair and makeup.

"Tali, you're *killing* me. Your patient is a hot mess!"

"Jeez, Irim. Why do you look like that at 7:00 a.m.? You're killing *me*. Anyway, come on, you can handle it. You love this stuff."

"*Fine*! You're right … I do."

I wink.

"Don't we both?"

DIAGRAM OF
THE PEDIATRIC AIRWAY

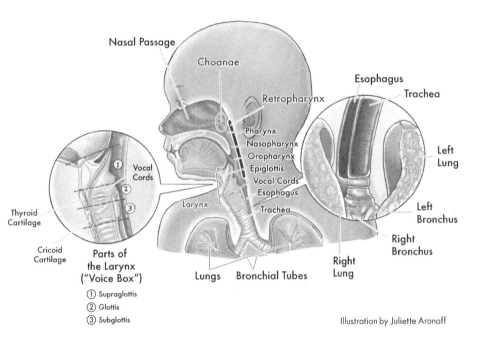

Nasal Passage

Choanae

Esophagus

Trachea

Retropharynx

Pharynx
Nasopharynx
Oropharynx
Epiglottis
Vocal Cords
Esophagus

Left
Lung

① Vocal
② Cords
③

Larynx

Trachea

Left
Bronchus

Thyroid
Cartilage

Right
Bronchus

Cricoid
Cartilage

Parts of
the Larynx
("Voice Box")

Lungs   Bronchial Tubes

Right
Lung

① Supraglottis
② Glottis
③ Subglottis

Illustration by Juliette Aronoff

CHAPTER 1

THE PREEMIE FROM THE PRISON

WHEN INFANTS ARE born extremely prematurely, they almost always require a prolonged period of mechanical ventilation. Their immature lungs can't function on their own because they weren't meant to. The main cause of this problem is the lack of a protective lubricating substance called surfactant. This substance helps the tiny sacks in a baby's lungs to inflate. When infants have a shortage of surfactant, they often require intubation. During intubation, a plastic tube is inserted into the trachea, the structure that is commonly known as "the windpipe." In ultra-premature babies, this period of intubation can last for months. Being intubated itself is not painful, but it is stimulating. Some of the typical medications used to keep patients calm have been shown to have deleterious effects on the brain development of neonates. To promote neurological development, the infants are *not* kept sedated. The tricky thing is that this essential tube can accidentally displace when the baby moves vigorously. These "self-extubations" can occur several times in these precarious first months of life.

The unintended consequence of these unplanned extubations is the formation of cysts. These cysts are caused by the chaffing phenomenon of the plastic against the delicate lining of the airway. This disrupts the fragile salivary glands dotting the upper respiratory tract. Once the tube is removed, a sign of the presence of these cysts is noisy breathing, either at baseline or only with illness. If the cysts are large, the infant can experience respiratory distress because the mucous sacks are occupying space. Often these young infants exist teetering on the brink of disaster. Unless they are sick or stressed, they may do ok. But, when they get into trouble, the decline is rapid. The key is predicting which way the situation is progressing and catching it before everything goes crashing downhill.

TIME-OUT

This is a 3.5-month-old, ex-25-week preemie who was found cyanotic (bluish/purplish) and unresponsive in the visitor's center of a maximum-security prison. Plan for today is to evaluate the airway and to perform any endoscopic interventions necessary to relieve the airway obstruction.

Patient Amari is a Day of Life (DOL) 102 ex-micro preemie who had been in the neonatal intensive care unit (NICU) at an outside hospital for her first three-plus months of existence. Like most ex-25-weekers, Amari was intubated at birth due to her inability to breathe spontaneously. She remained intubated until a month prior to discharge, when she transitioned to a less-invasive aid called positive pressure ventilation or continuous positive airway pressure

(CPAP). CPAP is the application of constant airway pressure through small tubes (nasal prongs) placed in the nostrils or a small mask around the nose. Instead of the machine controlling all respiration, the patient breathes in and out spontaneously. On CPAP, Amari did well. Her oxygen levels occasionally fluctuated with activity and position, but, in general, she maintained a reassuring baseline. Eventually, she graduated to breathing without any assistance.

Around that NICU graduation time, Jamila, Amari's mother, noticed that her baby's breath had a constant strange squeaking sound. Per Jamila's account, when she inquired repeatedly about this noise, she was told not to worry — that a doctor or nurse told her: "Premature babies just breathe that way sometimes."

Jamila is a Bronx-based woman in her mid-40s with an abundance of red-tipped, jet-black curly hair with stiletto-shaped multi-color acrylic nails and large gold hoop earrings. She has seven other children, most of whom are already grown. Two years prior to Amari's conception, Jamila underwent a tubal ligation. This procedure clearly failed because she nevertheless became pregnant with Amari, to her genuine surprise. The baby's father, whose name and extensive rap sheet I do not know, was recently incarcerated upstate. According to the prison's website, the visitor policy at that institution allows for up to three daily visitors and one child under the age of five, as long as the child is carried or sits on the adult's lap at all times.

On a frigid morning in mid-December, Jamila decided to take her newly discharged baby to meet the father for the first time. The baby's father was in a maximum-security prison that does not permit conjugal visits, so the conception timeline must have been tight. Perhaps that was what motivated Jamila to bring a tiny premature infant into the Family Visitation Center (FVC) on that fateful snowy day.

According to Jamila, prior to entering the Prisoner Visitation Center (PVC), all infants must first be stripped down to the bare minimum in the FVC. Then, they can be carried across the gravel-lined outdoor pathway that connects the two buildings. The distance between these structures is about a four-minute walk. I suspect the origin of this cruel-sounding policy emanated from previous attempts to smuggle weapons or drugs (or both) in the fluffy padded snowsuits of the innocent visiting babies. Admittedly though, that's just my conjecture.

Whatever the case may be, young Amari was dressed only in a flimsy cotton onesie and wrapped in a thin white receiving blanket when she was exposed to the freezing-cold air that day. Soon after entering her destination in the PVC, Jamila snagged the single available folding chair near the vending machine and began to warm up her daughter. It was at this point that she realized that Amari was limp and not breathing. Jamila started hysterically screaming for help. At this point, a heroic prison guard jumped over the barrier, grabbed the ashen baby and began performing CPR. Miraculously, Amari was successfully resuscitated. She was soon evacuated by helicopter ("helivaced") to our hospital. At the time of arrival, Amari was noted to be breathing laboriously, but on her own. Her core body temperature had returned to normal. She was admitted into the Emergency Department, Bay 32, with the diagnosis of "recent ALTE." An ALTE is an apparent life-threatening event in which the observer notes some combination of a pause in breathing, a color change, a loss of tone, or choking and gagging. In an infant, it's a near-death event.

As per protocol in these airway situations, our ENT team is alerted in advance of the patient's arrival. Therefore, my resident, Ann, is present at the initial evaluation. Upon examination, she notes deep suprasternal and abdominal retractions ("sinking in" of the area above the breastbone and stomach), nasal flaring, and head bobbing. All these signs indicate respiratory distress. The patient also has an audible high-pitched squeak on inhalation, called "inspiratory stridor," and a lower-toned sound on expiration, which indicates an increase in airway turbulence at or below the level of the voice box.

When Ann calls me, she sounds nervous, surrounded by the commotion of a loud and agitated mother and a crew of concerned transport and hospital personnel. I can tell she is unsure if the patient is stable or deteriorating. This is always a tough call if you don't have comparative data. A baby working harder than normal to breathe can remain stable for a while *if* that is their baseline and they have accommodated to it. On the other hand, a baby with sudden escalation in "work of breathing" can quickly tire out. Neither Ann nor I know Amari or her typical state at this point, so it's impossible to guess which direction she will go. Either way, I head in to help immediately.

In Children's OR 2, my team and I start preparing the necessary airway equipment in an efficient frenzy. All the relevant instruments are carried in. This includes an infant laryngoscopy tray, an infant rigid bronchoscopy tray, the microlaryngeal instruments tray, various rigid scopes, and a high-definition camera. I lay out the small-cup forceps in the most accessible spot. I organize the various-sized intubation tubes on my designated wheeling metal cart, first covering it with a paper sheet. The nurses run around in various directions, grabbing the disposable essentials: a clear-blue plastic tooth/gum guard (cut to size), a long-stemmed atomizer, 10 French suction tubing, and lens defog solution with a square absorbent sticky pad. Additionally, they obtain two medications: 1% lidocaine to topically numb the vocal cords and Afrin (a vasoconstrictor) to control any superficial bleeding. Minutes later, my harried resident bursts into the operating room, her dyed-blond hair spilling out from underneath her scrub cap. Despite her stress, Ann methodically surveys each element of the set-up just as I have taught her (good girl). Nevertheless, I perform a final "pre-flight-check" prior to green-lighting the patient's arrival.

Also present in the room (per my request/demand) are the "when all hell breaks loose" instruments — such as specialized airway balloons of various appropriate sizes — with the insufflator device primed and set to go. If all else fails, the open surgical airway tracheostomy tray remains at the ready on the nearby ring stand. When I'm concerned about a patient's well-being, I even open it up, to ward off the evil spirits. When I'm feeling confident, it's there in the corner with the plastic sterile seal left unbroken.

SURGERY START TIME — 6:43 P.M.

Amari is carried in by Dr. Bhupen Mehta. Bhupen is a soft-spoken, calm anesthesiologist of Indian descent who is board certified in both pediatric and cardiothoracic anesthesia. As a result, he deals with the sickest of the sick infants, so it takes an awful lot to rattle his chain. Even so, this baby is not making him happy. She is breathing but fighting like hell for each breath. Bhupen lays her gently on the operating table "cloud," as we lovingly call it. Technically, it's a Bair Hugger, a warm-air system that uses convective heat to prevent perioperative hypothermia, a particular risk in young infants. All the heart leads (wires) and oxygen sensors are then connected. In these tenuous airways, when the anesthesia begins, I demand total silence, shushing everyone like an old schoolmarm. All I want to hear is the steady beeping of the heart rate and the oxygen saturation monitor.

Each item I may use is arranged *exactly* so. Optimization is key before the unpredictable transition between wakefulness and anesthetic sleep begins. Bhupen has already begun his pre-oxygenation process. The patient's mouth and nose are covered with a small plastic mask as the sevoflurane gas flows through the long accordion-shaped tubing. This next point, Stage 2, is "the moment of truth." There are various stages of anesthesia, each with its distinct characteristics. Stage 2 is the rockiest period of excitement (e.g., involuntary movements, agitation) and airway reactivity. It is a period of disinhibition, tachycardia (fast heart rate), and delirium. Although the patient is asleep, their twitchy reflexes remain intact, so the airway is hypersensitive. These key minutes are the first test of how the baby will tolerate the procedure. I always instruct my residents to be vigilant during this time.

"Watch the chest."

"Observe the neck."

"Concentrate on the work of breathing."

"No chit chat."

"Focus *only* on the baby.

"Tune out everything else and everyone else around you. Listen closely to the monitor."[2]

It all begins ok. Her chest rises and falls appropriately, and the airway pressure remains stable.

Seconds later, the tide turns. Amari's lungs are no longer inflating with each squeeze of the bag. Bhupen faces increasing difficulty moving air. Mask-ventilation is no longer effective.

90 ... 80 ... 70 ... 60 ...

The baby's lips are drained of their healthy pinkish hue.

The pitch of the monitor drops into an ominous tenor.

"Beep . beep .. beep .. beep ... beep .... beep .... beep .... "

The heart rate begins to slow, a sign of impending cardiac arrest.

I take over control, quickly turning the bed 90 degrees coun-terclockwise "to the surgeon." A blue towel is wrapped around the baby's head to protect the upper face and eyes. A lighted laryngo-scope is hastily introduced into the right side "gutter" of the mouth to expose the airway below. A lens attached to a camera projects the image of the airway to the screens above. In place of a patent black hole, there is just a wall of pink. The immediate assumption is that the baby is in *laryngospasm*, a situation in which the vocal cords seize up in the closed position. But this seems unlikely, given the current depth of anesthesia in which the patient is totally relaxed.

---

2. My first cousin Michal was involved in a deadly home invasion in which a terrorist entered in disguise. In describing how she heroically protected her five children while the terrorist was in the kitchen, murdering her husband, father-in law, and sister-in law, she told me, "It was like a black screen came down on everything around me. All I could see were their faces. I knew exactly what I had to do to save them." In that critical moment, she gathered her twin babies who were sleep-ing in another room and her three other children and stealthily ushered them into a safe room. Although I would never equate Michal's harrowing experience to mine, it carries a lesson I take with me into the operating room. Whenever I am involved in an absolute airway emergency, I imagine a dark curtain lowering, ensconcing me alone with my patient.

In fact, the vocal cords are tethered shut. A thick white scar band is binding them together in a crisscross fashion.

There is only one move here ... intubate ... fast ... as atraumatically as possible.

The baby is gray-blue.

My eyes converge down the slotted metal barrel as I outstretch my hand and grasp the tube. It takes a firm screw-like maneuver to overcome the tension.

I know I'm in.

60 ... 70 ... 80 ... 90 ... 100

The escalating frequency of oxygen-monitor beeping is the reassurance we all need.

The entire room exhales.

Now that Amari is stabilized, it's finally time to fix her problem.

From a position of strength, I can comfortably remove the tube to quickly look inside the airway and figure out what exactly else is wrong.

On the first pass of the scope through the vocal cords, the problem is obvious. I identify multiple subglottic cysts blocking the hole. The largest one on the right sidewall is fluid-filled and occupies forty percent of the opening.

Ashley, my scrub nurse that day, intuitively holds out the micro-cup forceps. I unroof the biggest cyst with a grab-twist-yank motion, like uncapping a soft-boiled egg.

Viscous mucous oozes out satisfactorily as the cyst summarily deflates.

One problem is solved, but more problematic and posterior is that tight scar band. I need the laser.

The first application of the carbon dioxide laser for endoscopic surgery was in the 1970s by the intrepid surgeon Dr. Thomas G. Polanyi. The depth of penetration of the CO_2 laser is only 0.75 mm but it can still do a lot of damage, especially in the tight spaces of baby airways. Laser safety is taken extremely seriously in the OR, both for the patient and the staff. The concept of the dangerous "fire triad" is drilled into our brains: oxygen, heat, fuel. When these components are combined, combustion occurs. Fire in the airway is *bad*. We do everything to prevent it.

> The concept of the dangerous "fire triad" is drilled into our brains: oxygen, heat, fuel. When these components are combined, combustion occurs. Fire in the airway is *bad*.

First, we protect the patient.

Moist towels soaked in saline are used to cover every inch of the patient's face and neck. Then, the oxygen levels are lowered to the concentration of room air (which is not combustible). Everything in the surrounding area of the laser beam is also soaked in saline. Any conceivably flammable items are removed from the vicinity of the patient — except the essential intubation tube — until the last minute.

Second, we protect ourselves, specifically our vision. Special goggles are worn according to the laser's wavelength of light. The shades are pulled down on all in-looking doors or windows. Danger signs are taped to the outside doors, warning no one to enter. The laser is tested on a wooden tongue depressor to confirm that the red dot (the visible beam indicator) is aligned with the cutting action. The CO_2 laser is affixed to a special microscope, and a small joystick called a micromanipulator is used to control the beam. I look through the eyepieces, focusing the red dot on my target. Switching off standby mode, I step on the activation pedal.

The taut rubber-band like scar is gradually released as the laser beam slices through the thick tissue.

It is a tedious process, but effective.

At the last blow for freedom, her vocal cords finally spring open. Revealed beneath is the beautiful circular black hole of an open airway.

All is good. All is under control. Amari is okay.

The endoscopic surgery is complete.

The patient will be transported to the NICU in excellent condition.

Before I follow her isolette to the elevator, I glance back where the metal tracheostomy tray rests unopened. For today, the bright orange fastener remains intact.

DEBRIEF

"Prepare every last detail before the baby enters the room."

"Tune out the chatter."

"Check your equipment. Then, check it again."

"Be paranoid. Assume unintentional sabotage is behind every corner."

"Always remain vigilant. Trust no one."

"You are the surgeon. No matter what, in the end, everything is your responsibility. No one else's."

It may be irritating, but I instill these truths into my trainees like a Yogi's mantra. I'm sure when I turn my head, they roll their eyes like my kids do when I repeat myself for the thousandth time. But I don't care. It's one of the most valuable lessons I can teach them. I have no problem being known as the uptight asshole when it comes to my airway set-up. I want every tube styletted, every instrument laid out, even my special piece of clear-plastic one-inch tape for the head wrap must be placed to the left of my specific adjustable armed chair.

"FUCKING OCD Dr. Lando … again."

Call me any nickname … bring it on! For me, it must be the exact same way *every single time*. No substitutes, no exclusions. If the item is not in the drawer, go get it! If it's out of stock, order it! If you can't find something I need, search for it high and low. Others (including my more flexible colleagues) may be known as the "chill surgeons" — easy-going, improvising with whatever they're handed. I assuredly am not. And that's alright with me.

"Try to guess the most probable pathology, based on the information you know."

"Envision how you'll treat the problem."

"Run through the most likely scenario in your mind's eye. Then, the *second* most likely, just in case."

"When things go wrong (and often they do), adjust."

"Be agile like a ninja."

"In infant airways, you can never be sure what you are going to find."

"Have a Plan A, then a Plan B for when plan A fails, then a Plan C in case Plans A and B go to shit."

"The patient is counting on you. So are their parents."

"Ultimately, this baby's entire life rides on you. Deal with it or get out of the game."

AT HOME

My youngest daughter, Milla, was a preemie who spent two long months in the NICU at our local hospital after being delivered urgently due to my severe preeclampsia. Her birth was my first (but not last) foray into the other side of the medical experience. Though not requiring intubation, she needed CPAP immediately after birth to relieve her labored breathing. Milla's tiny eyes were initially covered with a spa-like mask as she lay in her isolette under the neon blue bilirubin lights. When my father first met her, he nervously joked that she looked like a space alien. Then he added, "At least now she has nowhere to go from here, but *up*."

My loving non-medical husband, Alex, peered at her through the plexiglass incubator with terror in his eyes. During that time, my head was flooded with all my patients' experiences: airway issues, brain bleeds, chronic lung disease, and developmental delays. Like many of the parents of my preemie patients, I stood at the bedside scared, helpless, and unsure of what the future would hold.

In many ways, Milla, Alex, and I escaped the NICU mostly unscathed. We didn't face the agonizing necessity of repeated surgeries or the long-term realities of bronchopulmonary dysplasia (under-developed preemie lungs). We were not the recipients of devastating news regarding abnormal head ultrasounds or troubling brain MRIs. The bigger challenges for our family played out in the years that followed, with neurodevelopmental hurdles. I've learned so much over the course of her beautiful and fascinating young life that it could undoubtedly fill the pages of an entire other book. But I'll leave her tale for another time.

All these years later, every time I enter the NICU with my residents to evaluate a baby, my memory still pings fresh to those vulnerable early days of Milla's life. Even as the expert consultant, I experience a visceral reaction to the sights and sounds of those tiny human patients encased in their plastic enclosures. Goosebumps erupt on my arms and the hairs on the back of my neck stand at attention. And, when I leave the unit, I always whisper softly to myself:

"I would much rather be the doctor than the parent any day."

All these years later, every time I enter the NICU with my residents to evaluate a baby, my memory still pings fresh to those vulnerable early days of Milla's life.

CHAPTER 2

THE LITTLE PERSON
WITH THE WIG

LIKE ANY WORKPLACE, ours has a colorful cast of characters and a unique culture. Despite our best intentions, immature arguments and petty squabbles periodically arise. Some days can get a bit thorny. At our core, though, we all swear by the same motto: "First, take care of the children." We instantaneously unite when patient care is at stake.

In addition to human nature, there are other barriers to the achievement of this lofty goal. Like many other hospitals across the country, we constantly face limitations in staffing, equipment, and physical space for operating. When it counts, though, our team jumps into action. I've seen it firsthand for pediatric head trauma, massive bleeding, and airway emergencies. It's truly a sight to behold.

In basic CPR, we learn the ABCs: airway, breathing, and circulation. The airway *always* comes first. That's why our job as pediatric otolaryngologists is so critical. We must establish the airway! Nothing is more important. Without breath, there is no life.

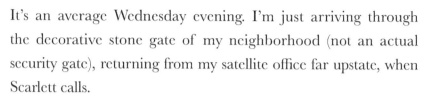

It's an average Wednesday evening. I'm just arriving through the decorative stone gate of my neighborhood (not an actual security gate), returning from my satellite office far upstate, when Scarlett calls.

"Mommy, where are you?"

"Almost pulling into the driveway, sweetheart. See you in five."

I'm about to hang up when I hear the long beep of the other line. It's Lianne.

"I am setting up the airway in Room One. The helicopter is landing in twenty-five minutes. I need you here. *Now*."

My esteemed colleague, Dr. Lianne de Serres, was once my attending (a fully trained doctor) when I was a mere first-year oto-laryngology resident at Columbia. She is the main reason I took this job. I can't imagine the last decade and a half without her as my stalwart friend. We talk frequently and have jointly weathered many professional crises, practice implosions, and other major life transitions. United together, we have gone up against "the man" in contract negotiations and, against great odds and surrounded by naysayers, emerged victorious. She is my constant sounding board and absolute port in the storm. Unlike me, Lianne is always put-together — she is the definition of cool, calm, and collected. She doesn't change her tone of voice or devolve her respectful disposition when stressed (like me). She is substantially more measured with staff and patient with residents (unlike me). Lianne is always reminding me, "They're just young, Tali. Give them a chance."

I call her MacGyver because she can jerry-rig any instrument to serve her purposes. But now, I hear the strain in her voice. This is serious.

Even though I will disappoint my daughter by disappearing back to work, I don't have a choice. I pull into the driveway quickly, throw the car into reverse, and back up onto the street once more. I turn right and race in the direction of the highway toward the medical center. Strategically, I live a mere eighteen minutes away, for situations like these — calls such as this, when there is just no extra time to spare.

When I arrive in the large semicircular driveway of the pediatric hospital, I screech to a halt and park illegally. I abandon my car near the huge bronze statue of a teddy bear sitting on what look like giant wooden blocks inscribed "A, B, C." I dart inside because every minute counts … because it's clearly that kind of emergency.

TIME-OUT (RUSHED)

This is a 2-year-old female who was crawling on the floor at home when she found and shoved a balloon in her mouth and inhaled suddenly and turned blue … and stayed that way. Parents called EMS, who brought her to the local hospital. They were able to maintain a life-compatible oxygen level with mask-bagging. She was flown here for airway foreign body removal, suspected to be in the trachea. Her neurological status is unknown.

Surgery Start Time — Immediate

Lianne has a case beginning next door, but she is ducking in and out of the room, helping to organize every element until I arrive. Seamlessly, I slide into the green leather ENT chair with the head of the operating table already rotated toward me (this is rare). Violating my cardinal rule, I only have time to eyeball the equipment.

Seconds later, a sweaty ER attending bursts into the room carrying a floppy, fully dressed toddler in his arms. The patient he hands me is a rag doll, pale and breathing shallow.

"Should I try to bag her up? Her oxygen levels are so low," says my anesthesiologist, Dr. Ashley Kelley.

I look her in the eyes and shake my head. Ashley is unflappable, even under pressure. She is a pretty, no-nonsense woman with long brown hair, blue eyes, and type 1 diabetes. She has two young kids and is married to a fellow anesthesiologist who I have never met (because he works constantly and because he's employed at another hospital).

"No time. Nasal cannula only. I gotta get it out or we won't be able to move enough air to make a difference."

There are too many people in the room: ER doctors, ICU physicians, other anesthesiologists, and a pediatric surgeon. The din of background conversation infuriates me.

But I am razor focused on the baby.

Despite all appearances, when the monitors are attached, the baby's oxygen levels are holding in the mid-70s (not terrible) and the heart rate remains steady.

I know I have one shot; it better count.

I open the baby's mouth, insert the tooth guard, grab the laryngoscope, and expose the larynx and the crisp white vocal cords.

I swipe the alligator optical grasping forceps that Lianne has neatly laid out for me. I don't have time for the standard protocol: take a look first to assess and then extract.

With my naked eye, peering into the depths of the trachea, I discern a vague outline.

I squint to see a crumpled pink balloon completely blocking the windpipe.

At this moment, I don't know how the child is alive.

With my left hand pulling upward in an angled trajectory, my right hand grasps the tip of the pink latex.

Pull … gently, gently.

Between the toothed metal tines of my instrument, I can feel the added weight of an object.

I retract my hand slowly, steadily, until the fuchsia rubber ball exits the trachea, crosses the narrow point of the subglottis, passes through the V-shaped aperture between the vocal cords, and then, finally, emerges out through the mouth.

I suspect the crowd erupts in cheer, but the room is a blur.

I remain fixated on the child, replacing the obstructing foreign body with a 4.5 cuffed endotracheal tube in one fluid motion.

"Intubated! Squeeze the bag. Bring her up. Squeeze the bag. Ventilate."

Ashley compresses the green reservoir bag repetitively as the precariously low oxygen levels begin to rise. Initially, we all sigh with sweet relief, but we soon notice the saturation numbers leveling off. We are not yet out of danger. Instead of the reassuring fog of condensation, pink frothy fluid bubbles up the intubation tube. Ashley and I know what's happening. It's the life-threatening post-obstructive pulmonary edema (**POPE**). POPE is the result of an abrupt shift of fluid into the lungs occurring shortly after clearing a severe upper airway obstruction.

As expected, Ashley is already prepared. She maintains positive pressure and pushes Lasix (a diuretic) into the IV line. It's tenuous at first, but over the next several minutes, the oxygen saturation climbs, reaching the high-80s. This is not yet normal. It's better, though, much better. The complete resolution of POPE will take a bit of time, management, and patience by our pediatric intensive care unit (PICU) team. But for now, we are out of the woods.

Regaining awareness of the world around me, I feel a hand on my shoulder.

"You did good."

It's Sam.

Butterflies. Exhale.

"Thanks … was a team effort."

"You did good though."

Double pat.

Ashley and my resident transport the patient to the ICU in stable condition. I set off in pursuit of the child's mother.

A few problems surface immediately. Halfway down the hallway, I realize that I don't even know the child's name. In these absolute emergency situations, patients are often given a genderless pseudonym. In the computer, this child is only listed as "Trauma Charlie."

Second obstacle, I don't know what her mother looks like … at all.

I double-back to the ER, in search of a nurse who might have some relevant information.

All I discover is that no one has seen her.

Apparently, the patient was flown in from the community hospital while the mother rode behind in an ambulance.

With some goading, the charge nurse calls out in a booming voice, "Anyone here who took care of Trauma Charlie?"

Non-contributory blank stares.

After a while, I finally identify a friendly clerk who *may* have caught a fleeting glimpse. She describes the mother as "a very short woman with a long skirt and a straight brown wig." No one has any clue where she disappeared to. In the fuzzy comedown from the adrenaline rush, I imagine myself chasing a tiny gypsy from a circus troupe with wild flowing hair and a bohemian-style dress. I wander the hallways aimlessly for at least fifteen minutes looking for someone matching that phantasmagorical description. Eventually, drained from all the backtracking and lack of success, I give up. I swipe my badge and climb the stairs to the second floor, checking the family waiting area on my way into the PICU.

Still, no tiny gypsy lady.

Inside, I scan the electronic tracking board and find my patient's room number.

"Trauma Charlie 3102."

When I enter, I spot a petite religious woman with a long black skirt and a brown wig (sheitel), swaying back and forth, mumbling. She is deeply engrossed in prayer.

I let out an audible chuckle.

That makes so much more sense.

She stops abruptly, and looks up at me, pleadingly.

"I took care of your daughter. She is safe. We got the object out. She will need to stay in the ICU intubated with a tube until her lungs recover. In the morning, we will order an MRI of the brain to see if there is any evidence of swelling from lack of oxygen. But I am hopeful that she will be ok."

"Baruch Hashem [Blessed be G-d]," she says.

And as I walk off the unit, I do thank Him too.

DEBRIEF

"Sometimes, it will come down to just you, and only you."

"Trust your abilities. Rely on your training. Remain calm. You can do this."

"When the stakes are high, do not panic."

"There is a reason you were accepted to this difficult field. Many apply, few get in and not everyone completes their residency."

"Even when you succeed, don't get distracted. There will be time to celebrate. In the immediate aftermath, do not let your guard down. Concentrate until the very end. Think of possible complications. Make sure your patient is totally in the clear before you pat yourself on the back and relax."

"Then, when it's a big win like this, make time to celebrate. Savor the moment. Breathe."

"You earned this! Really, you did."

AT HOME

I'm smiling on my drive home. I crank up the music, feeling a bit like a rock star. This euphoria is unlike any other: the direct act of saving someone's life. It's invigorating and addictive but it's also ephemeral. Most of the time, only the few people in the room really get it — how close of a call it was … how tenuous the life-and-death moment really was. It could have ended differently. Horribly.

This euphoria is unlike any other: the direct act of saving someone's life. It's invigorating and addictive but it's also ephemeral.

The summary to the parent often sounds matter of fact, implying that the medical "save" was routine:

"Everything went well. We were able to successfully [fill in the blank with procedure] …. Your child [enter name] is in the recovery room."

However, we few in that room grasp how close to the brink we came. Only we peered together over the abyss at the face of death and pulled that baby girl back toward life.

We know the win was so huge, because the loss would have been catastrophic.

So, yeah, I'm driving home and I'm flying high.

My window is wide open and I'm blasting P!nk.

"So raise your glass if you are wrong … In all the right ways …"

The song is so freakin' loud. I'm sure other cars next to me can hear every word, but I deserve this celebration.

"Won't you come on and come on and raise your glass … Just come on and come on and raise your glass …"

The world around me stops spinning for a while. I'm at the epicenter of the universe.

Despite the fanfare in my head, at the end of my brief trip home, everything will fade into absolute normalcy. The kitchen will be dirty, and the kids' homework will remain undone ... Dinner will be uneaten and PJs unadorned. Teeth will be unbrushed and bedtime stories unread. While I've been busy being Dr. Lando, my daughters have been waiting for Mommy.

Though I steal myself against the startling transition, I will soon experience all the typical frustrations wifely and motherly. And that's ok. It's normal.

Lean in and pay attention, though, for I have some wisdom to impart ...

Always ride the highs when you can ... because they are rare, merited, and short-lived.

You will see (and I already know from great personal experience), the lows can be rock bottom. No one knows what tomorrow will bring.

CHAPTER 3

HER NAME WAS JULIET, "WITH ONE T, NO E"

IN MEDICINE, AS in life, we are forced to make educated decisions in the present without knowing the impact of these choices in the future. All we have at our disposal to guide us is our intuition, years of intense residency and fellowship training (in my case, seven), followed by more years of hard-earned experience. We pepper in the advice of our mentors and colleagues and add the accessible wisdom from the vast medical literature.

When things go wrong, we torture ourselves with the clarity of hindsight, or at least I do. I wish I had a crystal ball to see every outcome of every intervention I perform, and those, like this one, that I did not perform. I wish my career as a physician was only filled with success stories and happy endings, but there are disappointments and tragedies too.

I wish for a lot of things but, mostly, I wish none of this story was true.

Juliet is an adorable baby with big brown eyes and curly auburn hair. On admission, she has a low-grade fever and a hard time swallowing her secretions. She had previously been in an outside hospital for two days with a viral illness and decreased oral intake. When she didn't improve, they started IV antibiotics. When she worsened still, they obtained CT imaging, which was suggestive of a "retropharyngeal phlegmon, no drainable abscess." A phlegmon is an ill-defined mass-like inflammatory process of the soft tissue. It is an early sign of infection deep within the neck. This finding prompted the doctors at the initial hospital to transfer her to our pediatric hospital around 9:30 p.m. on a Tuesday night.

Juliet is the first child born to two sweet, young parents. Her mom, Clarissa, speaks perfect English; her father does not. On arrival, Juliet is a bit sicker than the average patient with a similar diagnosis. Her heart rate is somewhat erratic, her breathing quickened, and her airway sounds wet, but she is not in any respiratory distress. Nonetheless, she is transferred to the Pediatric ICU for closer observation and medical management.

ENT is consulted. We suggest broader intravenous antibiotics to cover potential aggressive organisms, such as MRSA (methicillin-resistant Staphylococcus aureus — a type of antibiotic-resistant bacteria) and enterococcus. Over the next hours, Juliet continues to spike fevers. Upon examination, she whimpers whenever her head is tipped even slightly upward. This is suggestive of a retropharyngeal process (back of the throat problem), an entity we otolaryngologists encounter constantly because of its frequent occurrence in "our" region of the body. With the newer medication, Juliet fails to improve. So, by Wednesday afternoon, an updated CT scan of the neck is ordered. It is completed in the late evening, confirming progression to an abscess, a discrete drainable collection. As per standard protocol to limit radiation, the images only include the area in question, which is the neck to the level of the clavicles (collarbones).

The radiology report reads, "Rim enhancing lesion in the retropharynx suggestive of abscess. No notable extension into the chest. Further imaging of the chest may be obtained if indicated."

It is now 10:30 p.m. I am home. The non-pediatric on-call ENT attending rings me for advice.

"The OR is backed up with emergencies and this case wouldn't go until around 1:00 a.m. Is there any reason you think this baby needs to be taken to the operating room urgently in the middle of the night?"

"As long as she's stable clinically, it shouldn't make a difference to go first thing in the morning. When did she last eat?"

"The nurse said she just drank a bottle of formula, so we'd have to wait six hours anyway. It's only a few hours difference."

It is customary to avoid surgery on babies and young children in the middle of the night unless it is deemed an emergency. There are several reasons for this standard practice. First off, during the day, there is an excellent support system. If a patient is unstable, the anesthesiologist can easily call for help and a friendly colleague immediately runs in to assist. At night, there is limited back-up. Moreover, many hospitals (including ours) do not run the pediatric operating room 24 hours a day. After-hours cases go in the "main OR." Therefore, these cases are necessarily performed in subop-timal conditions, with a skeleton crew, out of the usual environ-ment with less accustomed staff. So too, we maintain restrictions on pre-operative eating (due to the risk of aspiration at the start of anesthesia) unless the case is declared an emergency. This is true even for babies.

We collectively decide to place the baby on the operative schedule for "first-start" at 7:00 a.m., which will be Thursday morning, before the scheduled OR cases are slated to begin. The covering surgeon is relieved. When we hang up, I nod off because I now have an extra early wake-up.

The next morning, I arrive at the PICU around 6:40 a.m. to evaluate the baby prior to her being transported to the OR. She has junky upper airway sounds. I open her mouth and depress her tongue. She cries, wretches, and immediately spits up a big glob of pus. An area in the back of her throat continues to drain murky yellow fluid. I obtain a culture. Five minutes later, her noisy breathing resolves completely.

"Wow! She sounds so much better," the baby's mom, Clarissa, notes with relief. "Please, doctor, since she is better, maybe she doesn't need surgery anymore. She's breathing normally again. Can we wait and see?"

She had not yet signed the surgical consent form.

I am skeptical. These deep infection pockets rarely open spontaneously. Most of the time, they require formal surgical drainage through the mouth. But spontaneous drainage *is* within the realm of possibility. Maybe it is safe to wait and see. I also agreed with her mom — she *did* sound so much better … and something did rupture during my examination.

I hang around for twenty minutes, chatting with the ICU attending. Then, I return to Juliet's room.

She is now sleeping, still quietly breathing and swallowing her secretions.

"I think we're ok to hold off for now. I will let her drink but not eat yet. We'll see how she does. I can always add her back to the schedule later today or tomorrow morning."

Things remain status quo that day and night. The PICU never calls me back. I spend the rest of my Thursday busily attending to my other surgical patients.

On Friday morning, I speak to my team and Juliet is still doing well. She's drinking her bottle, and her vitals have been basically stable. For the rest of the day, I am occupied with my clinic. By the evening, there are no changes when I check in.

Early Saturday afternoon, Juliet spikes another fever and appears lethargic. Both pediatric ENT and pediatric surgery are called to reassess. On meticulous re-read of the CT scan at the base of the neck, there is some concern regarding a tiny trail of downward-tracking fluid into the chest. However, the images are cut off at that point.

Retropharyngeal abscesses in children are rarely complicated by extension of the infection into the mediastinum, the space in the chest that holds the heart and other important vessels. It does happen, though. We've all seen it.

Samir, the general pediatric surgeon, and I meet up at the OR control desk to jointly book the case. My plan is to make an intraoral incision in the back of the throat to drain any remaining pus. His plan is to probe more inferiorly (lower) with the clamp to reach the upper chest.

TIME-OUT

This is an otherwise healthy 15-month-old female with a history of fevers, decreased oral intake, and neck stiffness caused by a retropharyngeal (the space located in the back of the throat) abscess

*here for intraoral incision and drainage by Dr. Lando (me), ENT,
and transoral upper mediastinal (chest) drainage by Dr. Pandya
(him), Pediatric Surgery.*

SURGERY START TIME — 2:30 P.M.

I start first, inserting the mouth gag and obtaining access to the back wall
of the throat. I make a vertical incision with the 15-blade knife near the
previous drainage site and cut through the thin mucosal lining of the
posterior pharyngeal wall. The incision is deepened through the underlying muscles. I use a tonsil clamp to open a substantial pocket between
the muscle and the fascia (the lining layer that encases the spine). Rather
than a rush of pus, barely anything comes out. This confirms the fact
that the abscess had already auto-drained two days prior. I irrigate the
wound anyway.

Samir takes over and extends the pocket deep into the upper
part of the chest. He irrigates the inferior cavity and only scant
purulence oozes out. As a precaution, he tucks in the catheter and
then snakes it along the back of the throat and through the nose.
This encourages any remaining pus to drain out. He stitches it
loosely in place.

Overall, the case is short, uneventful, and unsatisfying. We end
the procedure and transfer Juliet back to the PICU in good condition.

On Sunday morning, I receive an update that Juliet is doing
well. Later that day, although not on call, I stop by to see for myself.

When my girls were young, I often brought one of them with
me on weekend rounds. It relieved my guilt at leaving my husband
at home alone with all three kids. It also gave me a chance to
spend some special time with each of them. Lastly, it gave them

a glimpse into what Mommy does for a living, why I am gone so often, and for whom.

That day, I brought Juliette along. When we approach the large glass doors of the patient's room, I instruct her, "Juliette. Sit here and be a good girl for Mommy."

"What's that girl's name?"

"Actually, it's just like yours. Juliet, only with one T and no E."

"Can I meet her?"

"No, Juju, she's too sick."

I turn to walk inside. My Juliette sits on the nearby swivel chair, happily spinning.

Despite my warning, she immediately peers over the ledge, taps on the glass, and waves excitedly.

For the following several days, Juliet remains in the ICU on culture-driven (based on the samples of pus obtained) antibiotics. Her body seems to be responding, albeit slowly. Objective signs of infection — including her elevated white blood cell count and fever — decline appropriately. But the volatility of her heart rate persists. At my insistence, pediatric cardiology is consulted. After recording a normal EKG, they leave a note in the chart stating: "Tachycardia in the setting of infection. If it continues, consider obtaining an echocardiogram."

Everyone else seems to be relaxing. Yet, I can't shake the prickling feeling that something is still wrong. I contemplate ordering more scans to specifically include the chest, but this would be her third round of contrast radiation in a very short period.

It's a lot for her young kidneys. I consider getting an MRI, but it's typically more useful to compare the same imaging modalities (i.e., CT to CT or MRI to MRI, not CT to MRI). Moreover, the intensivist (the specialized physician who provides care for critically ill patients in settings like the ICU and PICU) and cardiologist are not concerned. It's just me and my gut.

I find myself hovering outside the door of our cardiothoracic surgeon.

Finally, I knock, and he waves me in.

"Sit, sit. What's on your mind?"

"Have you ever seen an infant with mediastinitis whose only abnormal vital sign is fluctuating tachycardia?"

"WBC, blood pressure, fever?"

"All normalized."

"No. I don't think it's possible. She'd be much sicker. There'd be other symptoms."

"Thanks."

I hesitate, then get up to leave, feeling slightly reassured.

After three more days of careful observation without any worsening, Juliet is downgraded from the ICU to the regular floor.

It's Monday at 6:35 p.m.

After finishing my cases in the OR, I round with my team.

We are on the third floor in one of the regular pediatric units dubbed "Superheroes."

When I emerge from a patient room, someone grabs my arm forcibly.

"Dr. Lando. Something is wrong with my baby."

Clarissa pulls me inside and points.

On the left side, at the base of Juliet's neck, just above the clavicle is a distinct abnormal bulge.

Something is very wrong with her baby.

"I will be right back."

I walk swiftly to the nearest computer console. In the order section, I type, "CT neck/chest with IV contrast." Under the priority section, I chose, "STAT."

I dial the radiology desk from my cell phone as I hurriedly take the stairs, two steps at a time, down to the pediatric OR desk, leaving my team bewildered.

"Hello. This is Dr. Lando. I need this scan to take full priority over any other imaging except absolute emergency head CTs."

Dr. Pandya's partner, Dr. Whitney McBride, is standing in the OR hallway. He has just completed his scheduled cases.

"Whitney, *please* don't leave the hospital."

He registers my anxiety.

"I won't. I promise."

A record-breaking 25 minutes later, my helpful resident, Annie, pushes little Juliet's stretcher into the scanner. I stand there, glued to the computer, waiting for the images to upload. When they finally do, it reveals exactly what I most feared. Whitney and I look at each other with dread. There is a large abscess cavity in the chest. There is nothing remarkable in the neck. We call Samir because he's the master of thoracoscopy, an endoscopic procedure to examine the chest. An endoscopy is a procedure that allows a physician to insert a medical tool through an opening in the body made with a small incision. A tiny camera with a light is inserted to see what's going on inside the body (as well as various surgical tools to fix the problem).

Without hesitation, Samir drives back to the hospital from home.

We have wheels into the OR at a stunning speed. It's less than two hours since Clarissa first grabbed me with that panicked look in her eyes about her baby's fate. That timeline from initial evaluation to radiographic diagnosis to surgical treatment is a truly astonishing feat.

TIME-OUT

This is a 15-month-old full-term infant who presented with a retropharyngeal abscess and was taken to the OR last week by myself and Dr. Pandya for intraoral and trans-cervical drainage. She is here again today for thoracoscopic drainage of a large chest abscess abutting the great vessels of the heart. **I am here as an observer.**

I sit silently on a stool, with my back against the wall. Dr. Pandya is *The Boss.* I watch the screens above, transfixed as he adeptly decompresses the main pocket noted on the imaging while navigating potential pitfalls. The abscess is situated in front of the aorta, a giant pulsating vessel coming off the heart. That isn't the only problem. The infection isn't contained. It's everywhere. The chest is filled with it. Samir spends hours working our small patient, painstakingly peeling purulent material from vital structures without causing any damage. He flushes the cavity with antibiotic irrigation. I just stay there, helplessly, silently. He completes a very thorough "debridement and washout." Eventually, he is finished.

Astonishingly, Juliet's vitals remain stable throughout the case. She loses minimal blood.

"Thank you, Samir. That was an amazing job."

"No problem. Glad you caught it. I really think she'll do well. Continue IV antibiotics. She may require a PICC line (a thin catheter used to provide long term antibiotics directly to the larger veins). Her body's immune system should take care of the rest."

She is transported upstairs while we go out to talk to the parents and relay the good news.

But over the next week, despite all our expectations, Juliet does *not* do well, not in the least. Her immune system does *not* take care of the rest. Not at all.

In contrast, her body deteriorates rapidly into full-blown multi-system organ failure. From initial hope, there is now only a descent into despair.

I wake up suddenly at 5:30 a.m. Monday morning.

Juliet's heart stops at 5:59 a.m. that same day.

None of it makes sense. The surgery was a success. Her cultures grew out MRSA that was specifically sensitive to the antibiotics she was already on. So, why did she still fail medical treatment so precipitously?

In the final report (which I obtained), Juliet's autopsy revealed a previously unknown, pre-existing, rare, life-threatening syndrome that can affect infants and children. In this situation, the immune system can be triggered by infection to act in a dysregulated manner, resulting in organ failure and death. This illness is rarely detected and identified in advance. These children appear healthy and robust, until they get really sick. On analysis of the literature, the correct diagnosis is only made premortem (before death) in one percent of such patients. Sadly, as in this case, the overall mortality rate is higher than eighty percent.

Her porcelain complexion and adorable smile were an immutable fact, but Juliet's picture of perfect health was an illusion.

DEBRIEF

Not surprisingly, Juliet's death flooded my mind with unanswerable questions.

What would have happened if I had taken her to the OR in the middle of the night, that first fateful day?

What if I had taken her early the next morning?

What if we had obtained that third CT scan — to include the chest — earlier?

Would it have made any difference in her outcome?

Was the cat already out of the bag from the start, evidenced by the enigmatic fluctuations in her heart rate?

Had the infection already spread by the time of transfer, her compromised and immature immune system incapable of containing it?

Or could I have stopped it?

Could I have saved her or was there never any hope?

The image of her cherubic face and pudgy cheeks rips at my heart as I stand at the lectern in our "Morbidity and Mortality" (M & M) conference to answer for my decisions. I present her case as objectively as I can.

"Dr. Lando, you couldn't have known."

But *should* I have anyway? Despite my best efforts, I lose my composure. Tears stream down my face.

When I call Dr. Mike Rutter, my professional touchstone and master of airway surgery, he gently reminds me what I need to hear again and again:

> "The patient is the one with the illness. Despite our best efforts, bad things can still happen, even to cute, innocent children with the same name as your daughter. You have to maintain faith that the good you bring to the world outweighs the occasional terrible outcomes. Not everything is in our control."

Hindsight may be 20/20, but foresight is murky and unclear. You can make the right decisions at the time with the information you have and it can still end badly. It is so easy to judge when looking back. Hindsight can torture you with self-doubt and regret. In the end, the best I can do is to take care of my other patients, learn from Juliet, and keep retelling her story to teach others.

Hindsight may be 20/20, but foresight
is murky and unclear.

"Carefully follow the trail of infection from the neck, downward. Confirm that it ends, then look again. Do *not* rely solely on the official report."

"Question symptoms that don't make sense. Look to the other teams around you and push them to do the same."

Still, all the lessons in the world can't bring Juliet back.

AT HOME

I arrive home late that cloudy night. I pull into the garage and sit in my car, long after the white vinyl overhead door has closed behind me, long after the automatic lights have shut off. I sit in the dark. When I finally peel myself off the leather seat, stand up, and go inside, the house is quiet. Even my dogs — who usually greet me effusively and loudly in the mudroom — do not stir. They must sense that tonight is not a time to awaken everyone with raucous barking.

Upstairs, I follow the glow of the nightlight into my Juliette's lavender bedroom. I crawl into her twin-over-full bunk bed, desperate to hear her steady breath. I watch her chest rise and fall and feel her regular heart beating until my pulse synchronizes with hers. Only then can I clear *her* image from my mind long enough to fall asleep. That precious baby girl is forever gone, with the same beautiful name as my daughter.

Tomorrow, I will wake up again, dress in my scrubs, string my ID badge around my neck, and start my day anew. But for Clarissa, I know life will never be the same. And even though there is no comparison between the depths of her loss and the grief I am feeling, I too will never be the same.

LATER

Sometimes, the story continues even when you are so sure it had a conclusive ending.

Two years later, a woman walks into my office with a young boy of 18 months. Immediately, I know her face and I note her last name. But the mother looking back at me does not register any familiarity. Even though she has come to see "Dr. Lando," a "pediatric ENT," she doesn't seem to know we have met before. I listen to her account of her son's sleep apnea. She describes all the familiar phrases — "long pauses in his breathing," "scary to watch all night," "snoring loudly and sleeping so fitfully," and "constantly congested." After numbing him with a spray, I pass my lighted scope through his nose and find the huge obstructing adenoid tissue. I recommend a simple surgical solution.

"It's a procedure called an adenoidectomy. Large adenoids are a very common problem for children of this age. I perform hundreds of these surgeries a year."

Looking at his sniffling and snorting — right now, while awake, mouth agape — I add, "He really needs this."

She lets me proceed. I recite the risks, benefits, and alternatives — as per protocol — as she listens calmly. I talk about recovery, scheduling, and day-of-surgery details.

Searching for the recognition in her eyes, but finding none, I continue.

I have to say it. Don't I?

I have no choice at this point.

"Mrs. Jones. Clarissa. It's me … Dr. Lando. Do you remember me?"

"No."

"I took care of Juliet. In the hospital, two years ago, in the ICU."

Her pupils grow wide. Still, she says nothing. I let the evanescent memory hang between us, suspended in time, afraid to break the spell.

"I cannot go back there. Not ever." Her voice rises angrily, "Do you *hear* me? NOT *EVER!*"

I'm holding my breath.

But she doesn't get up to leave, paralyzed by both the fear of doing nothing and the fear of doing something that could go wrong.

"I understand. I can help you. Let's find a place where you would feel comfortable. I'll call a colleague … anywhere you choose, in another hospital, in another area. I'll find someone wonderful who will take excellent care of your son."

To my shock and awe, she stays put, whispering almost imperceptibly, "No. It has to be you. It has to be *you* who takes care of him."

TIME-OUT

This is a two-year-old completely healthy boy here for an adenoid-ectomy for snoring and nasal obstruction. I will be using a coblator, as per usual. As a precaution, the oxygen will be lowered to room air throughout the procedure.

I perform nearly 400 adenoidectomies a year. In a young child, this surgery takes approximately five minutes for me to complete. I could practically do this in my sleep. Nonetheless, in atypical circumstances, there are special precautions to be taken. In a child with an unstable neck, I will maintain the child in a neutral position rather than extension. In a child with a bleeding disorder, I may have a special clotting agent in the room. If the bleeding issue is severe, I may even have blood products available just in case. In the most fragile of children — those with genetic disorders such as skeletal dysplasia or osteogenesis imperfecta (brittle bone syndrome) — I may even feel a twinge of nerves as I prop open the mouth gag and begin the procedure.

To say "I could do this in my sleep" is not an exaggeration.

But only in the rarest of rarest situations, those like this one, can I be overheard whispering a little prayer …

Let him be safe.

Twenty minutes later, after a smooth surgery and seamless anesthetic, I wheel a healthy boy into the recovery room.

Immediately afterward, I collect Clarissa from the waiting room where she sits rigid as a board, sandwiched next to her husband, sister, and mother.

"Everything went perfectly. There were no issues. He's great. Let me take you to him."

I lead her down the hallway, past the many curtains, to Spot 10.

I bring her back to her rainbow son.[3] He is tucked under the blanket, humidified oxygen blowing gently near his face, where he sleeps quietly, peacefully.

And just like that, he can finally breathe.

---

3. A "rainbow baby" is a common term for a baby born to a family after the previous loss of a child to miscarriage, stillbirth, or death from natural causes.

Juliet's jarring free-fall toward untimely death stood in stark contrast to the smooth post-surgical rebound of healthy patients like her brother. Though I turned to colleagues for support, the bulk of my torment played out privately, in the quiet recesses of my mind.

"Every surgeon carries within himself
a small cemetery, where from time to time
he goes to pray – a place of bitterness
and regret, where he must look for an
explanation for his failures."

———

FRENCH SURGEON HENRI MARIE RENÉ LERICHE

CHAPTER 4

THE ALGERIAN COUSINS

CONSANGUINITY — THE marriage of close relatives — is frowned upon in Western countries yet is common in many Middle Eastern cultures. The bint'amm marriage, or marriage with one's father's brother's daughter, is common — specifically in tribal and traditional Muslim communities, where men and women seldom meet potential spouses outside the extended family. Consanguineous marriages are estimated to be practiced by more than ten percent of the world's population, most frequently observed among families with unfavorable socioeconomic conditions. When these unions occur, they can pose a significant risk to their offspring. This is especially true in situations of autosomal recessive disorders, which require two damaged genes to come together (one from each parent) for the child to manifest the condition. Rare and often terrible genetic diseases are more likely to occur from the marriage of close relatives.

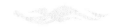

On a Tuesday morning, a woman — wearing a hijab and accompanied by her husband — comes into my office holding what appears to be an infant in her arms. On closer inspection, the infant is actually a three-year-old child who is extremely small for her age and severely malnourished. Through a translator, the mother explains that she has recently arrived in this country. The patient in her lap sounds terrible. Her name is Meriem. She weighs less than 30 pounds, is agitated, and is snorting and gasping constantly. I can't imagine how she coordinates breathing and eating, but from her gaunt appearance, I deduce that it's not well.

"Is this how she always breathes?"

"Sometimes, it's much, much worse."

The child is not verbal and recoils at my touch.

Meriem's father, Mohammed, tells me that he just managed to bring his wife, Fatma, and young daughter to the United States from Algeria.

When I ask if Meriem has any known diagnosis, Mohammed emphatically answers, "No." Later, he will admit that he didn't really know. When I delve further, I find out that Mohammed had immigrated to the U.S. first, leaving his pregnant wife behind in Algeria, and he was working in New York as a driver. He was already living in America several months prior to Meriem's birth, trying to raise enough money to bring the rest of the family over. He mentions that his wife, Fatma, did not always have access to fresh food and water or prenatal care during that time.

I scope Meriem and her entire nasal space is super tight. In the back of the nose, it should open widely into the nasopharynx and then gently angle vertically to the mouth below. The nasopharynx is the uppermost part of the pharynx (throat), located behind the nose and above the roof of the mouth. The thin 2.8-mm scope gets stuck. Eventually, I can manipulate a sharp turn through an oblique tiny hole, finally leading to the recognizable airway structures below.

I contemplate sending Meriem straight to the ER from my office. However, Fatma insists this is her baseline, so we agree to organize an intervention as soon as possible. In preparation, I order a thin-cut CT scan to specifically evaluate the bones of Meriem's skull. The imaging confirms my suspicion that the choanae, the two apertures at the back of the nasal cavity, are critically narrowed. It is at that point that I schedule her first surgery.

It's a Thursday morning when I park my grey Honda Pilot in the lot. On the way into the hospital, I bump into my anesthesia colleague, Kathy, in the parking garage.

"You gotta see this hilarious video of Hester with my dad."

I glance down to view her mix-breed dog and her semi-retired, widowed, dentist father "talking" to each other in short woofs and barks as if they are having a rational conversation about current events. I thoroughly love Kathy and her witty, snarky humor. We connect over our shared abnormal obsessions with our dogs and deep appreciation of sarcasm. She is also extremely capable, reliable in a crisis, and wonderful with children.

"Love it. Gotta run. See ya."

Once inside, I stop by the large whiteboard to see to which room and anesthesiologist I'm assigned. I trust the whole team implicitly. Still, each personality contributes to the tone and cadence (and sometimes even the length) of the day.

Room 2 / Dr Lando / Dr. Chan

Yes! It's going to be a great/efficient day. Dr Karmei Chan is a small but mighty Asian-American dynamo. Before joining our hospital, she worked in a non-academic center (without residents), so she learned to function like a one-woman show. Basically, she can intubate a child while simultaneously placing the IV and ripping the tape with her teeth to secure the whole thing down in one swift move.

"Tali, you ready?"

"Karmei ... you know I am ... always."

Time-Out

This is a 4-year-old blind, possibly deaf, female who recently arrived from Algeria with extreme failure to thrive and severe upper airway obstruction, here for endoscopic widening of her bilateral choanal stenosis.

These small choana (posterior nasal openings) can typically be widened using a combination of specialized pediatric sinus instruments, rigid scopes, and tiny drill bits. The only caveat is that the roof of these openings is the skull base, the bony encasement to the brain above. This is the immovable upper limit to creating this critical space.

Surgery Start Time — 9:00 a.m.

I insert the small rigid telescope in the left nostril to assess the opening.

"Urethral sound. Let's start with double zero, the smallest."

I sequentially dilate the space with larger and larger metal rods. Then I move on to the contralateral side.

"Small mushroom punch."

"Back-biter."

"Afrin-soaked pledgets."

"Suction."

The space quadruples in size from where I started, which is promising. At this point, I can't go higher because of the skull base, and I can't go more inferiorly either because of the bony part of the palate. I decide to end the case and see how little Meriem does.

Aside from some limitations in expansion, the case went as predicted. I turn Meriem back to the anesthesiologist.

One week later, when I see Meriem for follow-up, she is again very obstructed. In the office, I can see thick crusts at the surgical sites, which is expected. Despite twice daily saline rinses, there are copious nasal secretions.

I book her for a more comprehensive debridement in the OR and possible balloon dilation.

SURGERY START TIME — 8:00 A.M.

After suctioning out all the debris and peeling out the crusts, I find the bony openings to be slightly contracted, albeit still much wider than where I started.

"Insufflator."

I employ specialized 5-mm balloons to dilate each space a few more millimeters.

"Inflate up to 14 atmosphere."

"Set the clock for two minutes."

"Deflate."

I extract the balloons and suction the cavities.

The pictures I capture at the end of the case document the surgical success.

However, within days, it again becomes clear that Meriem's reality does not match those images. Her tumultuous breathing does *not* settle. Her feeding ability does *not* improve.

RETROSPECTION

When I brought Meriem into my operating room for that first attempt, I was filled with hope — hope that I would help her in some way. Regrettably, she didn't improve to the degree that I expected. I made some initial space in her tiny passageways, then I made some more. Over the next months, I returned to the operating room several times with Meriem to fight the battle. This is the norm in many of these cases. But even though I gained millimeters, it was never enough. I tackled the treatable risk factors for restenosis (reclosing), such as acid reflux, to no avail. Even though I knew it wasn't my fault, frustration set in.

I review the imaging with colleagues and conclude that the steep downward slope of the base of her skull is critically constricting the space. In theory, it too, can be drilled, but this is risky and can result in serious brain injury. Meriem sputters along, no worse, but no better. She ultimately requires a supplemental gastric tube to improve her nutrition, which was always critically impaired. She does poorly with illness. After repeated trips to the emergency room and admissions to the hospital for simple respiratory viruses, I have no choice but to bypass her narrow nasal airway altogether. I return to the operating room in defeat. This time, my goal is to create a surgical airway through her neck called a tracheostomy. Her parents do not hesitate to consent.

Meriem sputters along, no worse, but no better.

Once the trach is in, Meriem thrives. She is so relaxed now that she can breathe. When Mohammed is working, Fatma comes to the follow-up visits. On these occasions, she is always accompanied by her mother-in-law, a woman she introduces only as Nadia. I am impressed at how supportive Nadia is and how much she clearly loves this medically fragile child. She is unfazed by her granddaughter's plastic breathing tube, suctioning her gently when needed. On several occasions, Nadia even brings Meriem to the office by herself. Her visits continue at regular intervals every four to six months.

Later

One fall day, many years later, Fatma and Nadia appear in my office with Meriem and a cute three-month-old baby boy in tow. His name is Yousef. He is pudgy and smiling, tracking me with his huge black-brown eyes and long lashes. He looks perfect, sucking vigorously on his bottle. I am so happy for Fatma. She has begun to learn English and is adjusting well to life in America. She has solid family support.

"How exciting. Your first son."

"Yousef is not my first-born son," she confides in me.

"I did not know you had other children."

"I don't. But I once gave birth to a son who never took his first breath."

Within a month after that visit, in late December on a routine well-visit, Yousef's pediatrician notes that his soft spot is bulging. Mohammed then mentions that the baby's eyes are not focusing as before. Yousef is sent to the emergency room, where he is found to have hydrocephalus. Hydrocephalus is a condition where excess fluid builds up in the brain's ventricles, causing increased pressure. A CT scan of the head shows pansynostosis, the premature fusion of all the bones of the skull, creating critical compression of the brain. They run blood work. He also is found to have multiple metabolic abnormalities, including very low levels of calcium, magnesium, and vitamin D. Additionally, he has evidence of multiple fractures in his skeletal survey, with no known injuries. Yousef undergoes an urgent neurosurgical procedure to relieve the pressure on his brain. Although the surgery goes well, he subsequently develops difficulty feeding and a weak voice. The ENT team is consulted to evaluate his vocal cords.

When I walk into Yousef's room with my chief resident in consultation, I don't initially realize who he is. Then, I see Fatma and Mohammed look up at me, weary from the ordeal. I note their baby's involuntary eye movements and distinctly hoarse cry. I recognize that sinking feeling in the pit of my stomach.

After our laryngoscopic exam, we document "complete right vocal cord paralysis." Oddly, the new brain MRI does not provide any central explanation. I am baffled. What is causing these cranial nerve functions to fail? Nephrologists, neurologists, endocrinologists, and intensivists get involved, trying to piece together the enigma. A genetic panel is pending, but the parents report no family history of any such medical problems in their large extended family.

During his admission, Yousef endures many more tests and further imaging. More time passes, in which each symptom is treated as it arises. After weeks without a unifying diagnosis, the pediatric ophthalmologist, Dr. Kelly Ann Hutcheson, is consulted. In addition to the loss of his ability to track objects (from what was thought to be a neurologic impairment), Yousef's visual acuity is now deteriorating. In her consult note, Dr. Hutcheson writes plainly, "This is the classic ocular presentation of *infantile osteopetrosis (OPT)*."

After another major neurosurgical intervention, Yousef requires a blood transfusion due to critical anemia. This is the first time I can find in the medical record that the hematologist clearly documents, "The parents are first cousins."

As Yousef's vision dims even further, a risky hail-Mary procedure is attempted to save his sight. In conjunction with the neurosurgeons, a highly specialized skull-based surgeon is granted emergency privileges at our hospital to decompress the bony canals around Yousef's optic nerves.

Despite all efforts, Yousef continues to decline as his bones harden and thicken around his brain and cranial nerves. He undergoes a potentially curative bone-marrow transplant. His mother Fatma is the donor. After the exhaustion of heroic efforts to save his life, he is ultimately removed from cardiac and respiratory support, per his parents' request.

Posthumously, the results of more definitive genetic testing reveal an exceedingly rare recessive form of bony overgrowth disease that develops in infancy. Some of these babies are born completely normal and only develop symptoms when the skull bones start to prematurely close, encasing the brain under enormous pressure. Developmental progress halts and then the child regresses as he or she begins losing hearing and vision. Not surprisingly, when they also genetically test Meriem, she has the exact two defective genes, one from each parent.

DEBRIEF

It never occurred to me when I first met Mohammed and Fatma to ask if husband and wife were closely related. I had just assumed Meriem's condition was the unique result of poor nutrition and absent prenatal care, another innocent victim of a war-torn country. Here in the United States, it's just not a question you think to ask.

In speaking to my team about the case, I remind them …

"Pediatric patients always make sense eventually."

"Kids are only a mystery because we haven't figured them out yet."

"There will be a logical explanation. You just may not have deciphered the key code. Work hard to find it. When you do, a series of perplexing symptoms will become a unified syndrome. This may help you help the patient."

I had always sensed the closeness between mother and daughter-in-law. It struck me enough each time I saw them because it was so rare and special. I couldn't put my finger on why. In the end, it all became clear. Sadly, only Yousef's tragedy brought it into focus. Nadia was not only Fatma's mother-in-law, but she was her aunt as well.

AT HOME

The first time I met Fatma, I was a young attending, at the outset of my career. She was a recent immigrant, timid and unsure. She spoke no English and sat quietly and passively, with downcast eyes. I was so sure I could help her daughter. Though I never promised success, I was convinced I could create a sufficient nasal airway for Meriem to breathe comfortably. After all, that's what I was trained to do. A simple endoscopic intervention. Nothing fancy.

Little did I know what I was up against — her exceptional pathology and atypical anatomy. Her as-yet-undiagnosed disease beat me. After my first attempt in the operating room, I was humbled. After I brazenly tried again and again, I was tortured by non-fulfillment. But unlike me, Fatma adjusted. Her expectations were lower but realistic, whereas mine were lofty but ultimately unachievable. All I know is that she quickly learned to care for Meriem's "new normal." She mastered wound care, g-tube feeds, and tracheostomy tube changes and she weathered wound infections as they came.

I witnessed Fatma's evolution over several years of visits. I watched her confidence grow. I rooted for her. When she became pregnant with Yousef, I ignorantly assumed it would all be ok. And when I saw the fresh baby boy in the bright red carrier, I was truly hopeful for Fatma and her growing family.

Upon entering that hospital room years later, I never expected to see baby Yousef there. I never wanted to explain to his parents the connection between the vocal cord that was no longer moving and his deep brown eyes that could no longer focus. I didn't want to talk about nerves crushed by overgrowth of bone. I didn't want to hear their frightening rendition of a litany of "lost milestones." It seemed so unfair.

When I learned about the consanguinity, it was easy for me and others to judge. After all, genetic diversity is always the key to avoiding rare, inherited diseases. We all know that, don't we? It doesn't matter what country or culture you are from. Right?

When Yousef died months later, I was not in the hospital. Many more interventions had been attempted to save him. By then, our ENT team was no longer involved. I heard about his untimely demise by way of the pediatric neurosurgeon. At that point, many weeks had passed since his death. Despite my professional training, I didn't know what to say or do. And I am regretful to say that I did not reach out to his family at that time.

LATER STILL

I continue to care for Meriem and her airway.

I am distinctly uneasy about my first encounter with Fatma after Yousef's death. When I see Meriem's name on my busy clinic schedule that morning, I am on edge.

With each door I open, I peer nervously in to see if it's Fatma. *How will she be?*

What will I say? How can I comfort her?

Is it too late for "I'm sorry for your loss?"

How can anyone survive that grief?

I get so swept up in the day that I lower my guard. Around noon, I turn the knob to Room 4 and there she is. Meriem is on her lap, older but essentially unchanged. Nadia is there, too. Fatma's English has become fluent, and she responds articulately as I ask her my routine questions. But I cannot fathom the depth of the pain in her soul. Surprisingly, though, I do not sense it.

I force myself to look her straight in the eyes, to meet her wherever she is.

"I was so very sorry to hear about Yousef's death. There are no proper words. How have you been? Can I give you a hug?"

And she just nods, thankful for the recognition.

THE NON-EXISTENT DIAGNOSIS

"YOU JUST CAN'T make this stuff up."

We all love saying this. Dr. Mike Jacoby may love it the most. He is definitely the loudest pediatric anesthesiologist touting this phrase. Actually, he's just the loudest person in our surgery unit in general. Always upbeat and teeming with energy, with blue eyes and a boyish grin, the man doesn't have an indoor volume. We tease him constantly that he could wake up any patient from the depths of anesthesia with his booming voice alone. Still, I'd trust him with my own child any day.

Unlike Mike, I reserve this favored axiom — "You just can't make this stuff up" — only for the most unusual circumstances, when I am truly shocked by the peculiarity of medical reality. After all, most cases are straightforward and repetitive. The diagnosis is clear, and our treatment plan is almost reflexive. Most of the time, the symptoms are just as we learned about in medical school or residency. The truth is not as dramatic as the medical shows make it out to be.

This case was *THE* exception.

Every time I tried to understand it, I met another dead end. Every expert I asked gave me no usable feedback. No one could figure it out. I found myself repeatedly banging my head against a wall while faced with scared and frustrated parents, demanding answers that I could not provide. This case took me to the brink of insanity. But when I solved the puzzle (with the help of others), I experienced one of the most gratifying moments in my career.

Nathan is a full-term fraternal triplet who presented to our ER at 10 days of age, choking and sputtering. According to his parents, despite being a multiple, he had been doing well for his first week of life. He lives at home with his mother and father, new siblings, and one adopted older brother, Johnny. He has no known sick contacts. On the days leading up to his admission to the emergency room, he begins progressively gagging and making squeaky breathing noises. He has been hyperextending his neck and positioning himself at strange angles, especially when asleep, in a clear effort to open his airway.

The ENT team is called to perform a bedside flexible scope. I am the consultant attending at the time. My verbal description of the exam is not very technical.

"It looks like a bomb went off in there."

The entire surface of his larynx and opening to his esophagus is red, ulcerated, and swollen. There is a separate isolated lesion on the base of his tongue. It looks as if scalding liquid has been poured down there, or acid, or maybe boiling milk. My first thought is pretty dark. Did someone intentionally burn this baby's throat? Maybe it was accidental? I picture three new crying babies and a bleary-eyed parent, sleepily popping a bottle into the microwave out of desperation. Then, I imagine one baby yelping in pain and that same petrified parent calling 9-1-1. If not that, then what? Another sinister theory emerged. What about the 13-year-old adopted sibling, Johnny? He had lived happily for over a decade as an only child and now there are triplets! Could he have been jealous enough to swap the milk with something poisonous like a cleaning product?

There must be an answer. We will keep Nathan until we figure it out. First, we need a biopsy.

TIME-OUT

This is an 11-day-old triplet male with cyclical periods of respiratory distress and inability to feed of unknown etiology, who is here for a complete airway evaluation and tissue biopsy.

On first impression, Nathan's family seems normal, caring, cohesive, and appropriately concerned.

Mom shows me her screen saver. It's Johnny on the couch, grinning widely, wearing his "Big Brother x 3" t-shirt with three little bundles propped on his lap. Still, looks can be deceiving no matter how adorable the family. Above all else, we need to protect Nathan. At this point, we have no other answers. Later, when directly questioned (by child protective services), Dad calmly produced a picture of three Medela-brand yellow bottle warmers, side by side on the kitchen counter.

SURGERY START TIME — 12:25 P.M.

Surprisingly, the operative evaluation is uneventful. The mucosal lining looks terrible. I swab the laryngeal surfaces in multiple locations and send off a host of cultures: viral, bacterial, and fungal. I even obtain a specialized culture media from the Centers for Disease Control and Prevention (CDC) for diphtheria, a rare bacterial disease that can cause the formation of a thick, gray coating of the throat called a "pseudomembrane."

Similar to the "twist and yank" motion I use for unroofing a cyst, there is a modified "grab and pull" maneuver that is typically used to obtain a biopsy. In this case, it is essential to obtain a full-thickness sample that will enable the pathologist to examine all three layers in detail: mucosa, basement membrane, and underlying muscle. However, when I attempt to gently grab, the airway lining just shears. It is like pulling apart a piece of wet tissue paper.

Post-op, we admit Nathan to the PICU, place a feeding tube, and observe closely. Steroids and reflux medications are started to calm down the inflammation. Other organ systems are checked for abnormalities. A comprehensive renal evaluation reveals a defect in the drainage system of the left kidney. My team repeats bedside scope exams daily. If it is a caustic (intentional) ingestion, it should evolve in a certain way. Over the next several days, there are some changes in the findings. The ulcerations become less red and more fibrinous, and the secretions become thicker and harder to manage. Then, a strange thing happens. On days five and six, the mucosa starts to heal, turns pink, and almost appears normal. Nathan's constantly awkward, arched posture relaxes ... as does his breathing. When we look up at the video screen together, I see Mom smile for the first time.

On day seven, Nathan's brother, Justin, arrives in our emergency department in distress. When I hear the news, I am coincidentally at Nathan's bedside. Per the nurse, Mom had just gone home the previous night to shower, rest, and repack.

Upon ENT evaluation, Justin's initial exam looks strikingly similar to that of his brother, with two notable exceptions: the mucosal surface is more scarred than ulcerative and he has a skip lesion (separate area) on his gums rather than his tongue. Although Justin is later to the game, he leapfrogs over his brother in severity and deteriorates rapidly. Initially noted to sound "squeaky and wet," he soon requires intubation and mechanical ventilation. His echocardiogram identifies an abnormal mitral valve in his heart.

The baby brothers are admitted in adjacent rooms in the pediatric ICU. The parents frantically trade off shifts, keeping vigil at the boys' bedsides.

What the hell is going on?

Newborn fraternal siblings with some unknown, similar disease process — with different phenotypes (physical findings), no recent illness, or family history of genetic disease. And I checked … these parents are *not* close relatives.

We all assume that the third baby, a sister, will show up any day.

Though it takes another two weeks for final results, the cultures and biopsies don't shed any light on the problem.

"No growth — bacterial or fungal — and negative (normal) viral serologies."

"Evidence of superficial scarring and epithelium poorly attached to the basement membrane."

"No pathognomonic microscopic features for a known disease entity."

The only thing I keep circling back to is this skin-scarring disease I had learned about in medical school. This condition is part of a group of rare autoimmune disorders in which the body attacks itself. Maybe these babies both have the disease, but it is only manifesting in an isolated area of the body? There is only one problem with this theory: the body doesn't form its own antibodies until at least six weeks of age. These babies had problems way younger than that. Could there be a version of this disease that is even rarer and that *does* present at birth?

Turns out, the neonatal scarring disease can only occur in the first weeks of life if the mom transmits her antibodies into the baby's bloodstream. In that case, the mom also must have the disease. Nathan and Justin's mom did not. Also, what about the sister? She didn't have anything wrong with her.

Another impasse. Still, no diagnosis and no path forward.

Every day, I return to the brothers' bedsides — baffled, re-evaluating, re-examining. I am left with only questions, never answers.

I am left with only questions, never answers.

Even though the sister hasn't appeared, we all begin to knowingly refer to them as "*the triplets.*"

At home after hours, I scour the internet. For weeks, my nightly search history reads: "mucosal," "larynx," "ulcerations," "isolated," "congenital," "infant" — but at least one key term is always crossed out with a thick black line.

No exact hits.

In desperation, I call the pathology lab and force them to run a special stain for antibodies to the basement membrane, even though they tell me it isn't possible.

Infectious, environmental, and immune etiologies are all ruled out.

I keep coming back to genetics.

In this case, the parents are *definitely* unrelated, even distantly. Dad is from Chile and mom's family is second-generation American with Italian and Greek origins. They aren't even from adjacent continents. The chance of a new (de novo) spontaneous (not inherited) genetic mutation occurring in two non-identical siblings is exceedingly low. So low, in fact, that it is considered nearly impossible. Plus, the third sibling has no issues at all! So far, I have never met her.

Genetic reports are regarded as particularly sensitive material with built-in limitations in access. Therefore, as a non-geneticist, it can be difficult to find the results easily in the medical record system at our hospital.

After weeks of pestering, I was finally assured by the rounding hospitalist: "The genetics came back essentially normal." Still, I could not find anyone to show me the actual report.

The two babies kept getting sicker, then better, sicker again, then better again. Justin is finally extubated but still requires constant respiratory support. He is unable to coordinate breathing and eating by mouth. The parents grow angry and began insisting they be discharged because, in their words, "You don't know what's wrong with them and you definitely aren't helping them anyway."

I just couldn't let them go home like this. Not when they were this vulnerable ... especially Justin.

I had reached the logical conclusion. The entire multidisciplinary team agreed.

"I think we need to place a surgical airway for safety. Hopefully it will be temporary."

The parents refuse consent with every fiber of their beings. We meet with the entire team on multiple occasions but cannot convince them. Over the next week, though the babies' conditions wax and wane, they are overall stable from a breathing perspective. At the family's resolute insistence, Nathan and Justin are discharged home with no diagnosis and, from my perspective, no contingency plan ...

The first time I'm called to the emergency room in a panic, I am driving to pick up my daughter's bat mitzvah dress. As per usual, it is a Thursday evening. The bat mitzvah is Friday (the next day), so it is the absolute last chance to make alterations. My sweet daughter is sitting patiently in the back seat of the car. Our ENT physician assistant (PA) is at the bedside.

"It's one of *the triplets*. The ED tried to intubate, but they can't. They are trying again."

"Should I come? Can they do it? Is it the third one? The girl?"

"I can't tell. There are so many people. It doesn't look good. Someone is starting chest compressions."

I make a sharp U-turn, trying to punch in the hospital address to my GPS. I'm in an unfamiliar neighborhood and the rain is hammering at my windshield. I make a few wrong turns, stopping and starting, slowing, then speeding up. The visibility is poor.

Eventually, I get my bearings.

"What's happening?"

"Anesthesia is here."

Then the police lights flash behind me.

"Pull over," a voice booms over the megaphone.

I can't decide what to do. I pull aside, but I don't get off the phone.

"They're still trying to intubate."

I roll down my window, but I refuse to hang up.

"Officer. Give me one minute. It's a baby … emergency." I flash my hospital ID.

"Can they intubate? Did they? Answer me."

The angry officer waits impatiently. I motion to the cop to be quiet, then a pleading sign as I bring my hands together. After what feels like forever, my PA finally proclaims, "Dr. Murphy did it. She did it. The baby is intubated. Sats are coming up."

That was the first of such calls, but not the last.

The second one comes a month later and is just as heart-pounding.

This time, my phone rings at midnight on a night I was again not on call. I am in my pajamas with my blond-coated golden-doodle, Junie, snoring gently at my feet. When I see the number flashing, I know it is urgent. It's Dr. Rescoe, one of the pediatric intensivists.

"Come now," she says. "It's one of *the triplets.*"

By the time I arrive in the trauma bay, it's utter chaos. I weave my way through the sea of people straight toward the head of the bed where the baby is gasping and struggling. Mom and grandma are standing outside the door, crying. Mom tugs the corner of my jacket on my way inside.

"Tell me it will be ok."

I don't answer.

It was a shit-hitting-the-fan moment, but that's the kind we're trained for. You have to just shove others aside, take control, and be firm but calm. I remind myself, "I know this airway."

Find the hole. Eye on the prize ... Find the hole. Eye on the prize.

I hear the mom screaming now, "Tell me it will be ok. Tell me he will be ok."

When the tube successfully sneaks past all the abnormal scar and sloughed surface into the trachea and the carbon dioxide indicator turns from purple to yellow, I know I'm good. The blue baby turns pink. After the tube is secured, I slink back out through the crowd, past the mom who cannot meet my eyes.

Emotionally drained, I mumble, "He's ok now."

The next day, we place Justin's tracheostomy tube with mom's consent.

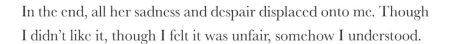

In the end, all her sadness and despair displaced onto me. Though I didn't like it, though I felt it was unfair, somehow I understood.

Three perfect babies — two with this horrible, incurable, undi-agnosable disease. In their anguished minds, someone had to be blamed. I was a convenient target. I was there.

I asked my trusted colleague to follow Justin until his hospital discharge. After that, the babies remained safely managed within my practice but just not directly under my care. That was the parents' choice, and I accepted it.

One month later, I received a call from *the triplets'* pediatrician.

"I have two of the triplets in my office. Did you see their genetic report?"

"I was always assured it was 'normal.'"

"Well, I am looking right at it, and it says, 'small chromo-somal deletion involving two genes of unknown significance' (i.e., they are missing specific genetic material and we're not sure what that means) …"

"And Tali … it is the exact same for both babies."

"What gene exactly?"

She tells me and I type furiously into the PubMed search engine.

What I discover solves the entire mystery. Their faulty gene codes for a specific protein involved in scar formation in the mucosal lining. It is most highly concentrated in the larynx (the throat).

Mic drop. Eureka. We found it!

**I type furiously into the PubMed search engine.
What I discover solves the entire mystery.**

DEBRIEF

This case is about the search for answers and the reason it took so long to find the truth. On a more personal level, it is about the unqualified belief that you have done everything in your power to help a child and the reality that a family may still lose faith in your abilities. The search in this case consumed me. I racked my brain, trying to solve the puzzle. Though I recognize that my challenge paled in comparison to their parents, the lack of an explanation still tortured me. There was something about these beautiful, healthy-appearing babies, drowning in their own secretions ... I wanted answers, not just for them, not just for the distraught parents, but for me, too.

Prior to the genetic discovery, I presented these infants in our multi-institutional complex pediatric airway conference. The response was throat clearing and the sound of crickets. I picked the brain of anyone who would listen to their convoluted tale. I scoured research studies for guidance. No one had a clue.

After processing their results, on the deepest dive into the medical literature performed by my diligent resident Rocco, we found one human case of a somewhat similar mutation and one case in a mouse model.

I wish I could say that this genetic finding clarified the trajectory for these kids, but it didn't. A disease that predisposes to scar is difficult to predict. In the end, the truth was just as agonizing as the not-knowing. Their clinical course was murky. Would they do better as their tiny airways grew? What about their overall development? It was uncharted territory, a place where no parent ever wants to be. But there are medical advances every day, especially in the field of genetic engineering. And I will continue to hold out hope for their future, monitoring their progress, even if it's just from afar.

In the end, the truth was just as agonizing as the not-knowing.

AT HOME

Lianne, with her quick wit and endearing Southern charm, uses a phrase called "drop-and-go emergencies." It perfectly encapsulates this specific situation in which minutes are of the essence. When you care for these airway kids, you must be ready to get to the hospital ASAP. To take this on is a choice you need to make deliberately in your career, because it will reach its tentacles into your personal life and try to squeeze it in so many insidious ways.

My daughter Scarlett plays basketball. I split some of the late practice pickup with a few other busy working moms. Her super close friend Meira's mother is a pediatric dentist and her bestie Nava's mother is a corporate lawyer. I've already called in countless favors for last-minute switches, so today *is* my turn. The school gym has a back entrance where I typically park my car. Frustratingly, the school is in an area near the Long Island Sound with a black hole of cell reception. I'm not a conspiracy theorist but I'm still convinced there's a hidden GPS tracker in my car that detects my arrival. The minute I enter school property is always the exact same

moment when I'm called back for some emergency. It's Tuesday
night when my phone rings. I see it's a hospital extension. On the
line, I hear a glitchy voice,

"Doctor … where … you … near … hospital … patient …
problem … nut … airway …"

Whatever the caller is saying doesn't sound good. Per usual,
I'm running twenty minutes late due to ten "just one more thing(s)"
from my medical assistant. Scarlett has already called me multiple
times for an ETA.

When I pull up, aside from my daughter, I see two other
7th-grade girls in red-and-white basketball uniforms standing in
the parking lot with wind-blown hair. The three of them are tired,
bedraggled, and clearly annoyed. I motion them inside and bring
my finger to my lips, requesting quiet.

"But, Mommy, I just need to tell you something."

I've already dialed back the OR front desk as I careen
out the gate.

"Hey, it's Dr. Lando. I think Dr. Tara Doherty just called me."

"Yes, she's in Room 1 already. They just rushed down
the patient."

Shit. That's not good. Tara is an excellent intubator. She's super
competent and she is not an alarmist either. It's already 7:00 p.m.
and the only reason they'd be in there is a *real* emergency.

Tara gets on the phone.

"Where are you?"

"In Mamaroneck, driving a carpool."

"How soon can you get here?"

"I have three 11-year-old kids in the car. Do I have time to
drop them off?"

"I don't think so. I'm bagging the baby, but this isn't a sustainable situation. If I tube her, I risk pushing the object further in, causing complete airway obstruction."

Then we'll really be screwed.

"I will be there in fifteen minutes."

I hang up and dial my husband, who is at an ice rink, at another daughter's sports practice. He also has terrible reception.

"I need you to leave there; drive to the children's hospital; double park in the front; pick up Scarlett, Meira, and Nava; drive them home; and then go back to the rink to grab Juliette. Gotta run."

Silent groan, then acceptance because he knows the drill by heart.

"Ok. Got it."

Forgetting all three jackets despite the freezing temperatures, I rush inside, hastily stranding the girls near the fish tank in the hospital lobby. I point to curvy orange pleather couches.

"Wait there. Be good."

I kiss Scarlett on the head, abandoning her and her thirsty, bewildered friends.

"Daddy will be here soon ... I hope."

"But Mommy ..."

I'm already way down the hallway when I realize that I left them to fend for themselves sans money or their water bottles.

When I arrive in OR 1, Tara is at the head of the bed, holding the mask, and her resident is squeezing the bag with two hands ... pretty hard. The oxygen levels are dipping deep into the 70s then rising up briefly, then dropping again. Something sizable is blocking part of the airway. Miraculously, Orlando, the OR desk head nurse, has stayed late. All the airway equipment is in the room, at least partially set up.

I'm just in time. It's the moment of truth.

I take over, positioning myself appropriately.

Left hand exposes, right hand reaches in.

The child's lips are a deep color of purple.

In these moments, if I'm not cursing like a drunken sailor, I am often talking to myself.

"Slow and steady pull. Do not drop it. Slow and steady pull. Do not fail."

I get hold of the object.

"Emerging intact from the trachea to the mouth and out."

The image on the screen transforms into reality.

"Boo yaa, it's a whole cashew! And it's *outta there* ..."

Whether it's the rare triplets or the many aspirated-nut kids, that's how it gets done. It's the sudden and inconvenient timing that disrupts everything. But as I said, I live 7.3 miles from the hospital as the crow flies for a reason. This job may leave a giant mess in its wake ... three cold, tired kids with their backpacks waiting in the cavernous hospital lobby ... repeated missed dental appointments until my cavity-turned-root-canal-turned-tooth-extraction becomes a $5,000 dental implant ... missed haircuts and color with unruly, unwanted roots poking through. There are never-ending schedule screw-ups, forgotten special-education Zoom meetings with the district, skipped parent-teacher conferences, forever lateness, and constant begging for forgiveness from everyone in my life.

It sounds like complaining, but it's absolutely the path I have chosen. The intensity, the necessity, being the go-to airway gal — that's what fuels my engines. I wouldn't have it any other way.

To paraphrase Cyrus Beene in my favorite episode of Shonda Rhimes's *Scandal,* "It's my hallelujah, heroin, and reason to live."

And truly, it is.

THE INEXPLICABLE OUTCOME

THERE ARE CASES that you do routinely and those that you do because they are a required part of your specialty's repertoire. Then, there are the select surgeries you really *love* to do. For me, the "ansa to recurrent laryngeal nerve anastomosis surgery" is the latter. The concept is this: an essential nerve has been damaged during a heart surgery or chest surgery (often in early infancy). The nerve function cannot be restored. A non-essential branch of another nerve can be swung around and stitched to the severed nerve. Power is restored to the nerve (like turning back on the electricity), but not natural function. The surgical technique involves the formation of a connection between the main stump of the damaged nerve and a branch of another intact nerve. This leads to reinnervation (return of power) of both the abductor (opener) and adductor (closing) muscle groups of the voice box. The surgery is ideal in its simplicity while intricate enough to require high-level fellowship skill. In the 1980s, Dr. RL Crumley was the first to describe ansa cervicalis to recurrent laryngeal nerve neurorrhaphy (nerve joining) as a treatment option in children. It is considered a relatively safe procedure with great potential benefit to the patient.

I was taught this surgical technique in my second year of pediatric airway fellowship. At the time, only a handful of surgeons in the United States were doing it in kids, although it had been long employed in the adult population. Because the indication is somewhat uncommon and the number of surgeons performing it at the time was limited, I filed it in my mind under the proud category of "my special skills." As a young attending, I performed it several times with great success in improving both voice and breathing outcomes (it can sometimes improve swallowing function as well). One of the most common reasons this procedure is needed is following ligation (closing off) of a heart vessel called the ductus arteriosus (DA) in premature infants.

The ductus arteriosus (DA) is a small artery that is open in utero to allow blood to bypass the non-functioning fetal lungs. It is supposed to close spontaneously at or soon after birth. Ninety percent of these arteries close by the eighth week of life, but in very premature infants (born at less than 25 weeks gestational age), many do not. If it does not close, it is referred to as a patent ductus-arteriosus (PDA). The persistent opening puts a strain on these young hearts, necessitating surgical closure. A well-known risk of this cardiac intervention is left vocal cord weakness or paralysis. The paralysis is caused by an injury to a nerve that loops behind the DA and then ascends to the larynx (voice box) to control the movement of the left vocal cord. This nerve is called the recurrent laryngeal nerve (RLN). Unilateral vocal cord paralysis can have a significant negative impact on the patient's quality of life in terms of their breathing, voice, and ability to swallow properly. Although surgical techniques are being continuously refined to avoid it, inadvertent injury to the left RLN still occurs.

TIME-OUT

This is a 2.5-year-old ex-23-week quad preemie with a known left vocal cord paralysis and breathy dysphonia (abnormal voice) from a previous PDA ligation. She is here today for a left ansa to recurrent laryngeal nerve anastomosis. The left side of the neck is clearly marked in blue. This marking was completed in the preoperative holding area.

Nina is a spunky little toddler with stick-straight brown hair and adorable small features. She has this comfort lovie, a gray rabbit that she keeps in her mouth like a pacifier, always shoved so deeply down her throat that it is a miracle she doesn't choke. Nina — nicknamed "Nini" — is a quadruplet, born at 23 weeks' gestation to wonderful parents, Lisa and Ron. Nina has one sister (Ella), one surviving brother (Gabriel, who has mild cerebral palsy), and one brother who had died at birth. At more than two years old now, Nina is sharp as a tack. At her initial visit, she has a quiet, breathy voice. When she tries to project, her neck veins bulge from the effort. She needs multiple breaks when speaking a sentence.

After her PDA ligation in early infancy, she had abnormal swallow function and was aspirating liquids into her lungs. Initially, she was fed through a nasogastric tube in the NICU. As she grew, she became able to tolerate thickened liquids but continued to have trouble with regular, thin liquids. Prior to our encounter, she had been followed by one of my colleagues, who noted an isolated left vocal-cord paralysis on multiple documented laryngoscopic exams. Nina also has inspiratory stridor (noisy breathing) with exertion and a tough time tolerating upper respiratory illnesses. She was referred to me for consideration of surgery to improve her voice and communication ability.

In the office, I note the same left-cord paralysis with contrasting right-sided cord movement. At this point, I think she's an ideal candidate for non-selective laryngeal reinnervation. A surgical date is selected — exactly three months from the Wednesday afternoon that she first skipped into my clinic. My trusted laryngology partner and I book the case jointly to combine our surgical expertise.

SURGERY START TIME — 8:00 A.M.

After an uneventful intubation, Nina is positioned with her neck extended with a standard-thickness shoulder roll and turned slightly to the right to expose her left side. Numbing medicine is injected into the future incision site and the neck is prepped and draped in the usual sterile fashion …

The case proceeds perfectly, just as planned. Her nerve location is "textbook." The rest of her anatomy appears pristine. The main stump of the injured left RLN is identified as expected in the tracheoesophageal groove at its entry point into the larynx at the cartilaginous cricoarytenoid joint. (I know, I know it's a lot of medical terminology but basically the nerve was where it belongs). The wispy nerve is traced downward delicately. The ansa cervicalis nerve is located anterior (in front of) to the internal jugular vein. The longest branch of the nerve is selected. In this case, it is the nerve to one of the "strap" muscles of the neck, known as the sternohyoid muscle. On a green rubber background, under the magnification of a high-power neurosurgical microscope, the two nerve endings are joined with several tiny 0.3-mm black nylon sutures. A special nerve wrap is used to prevent any aberrant connections from forming. The muscle and skin layers are closed in sequence. My colleague and I are both delighted with the procedure. Nina is turned back to anesthesia for awakening and extubating.

As soon as the tube is removed, she struggles. Her neck muscles tighten, and she has loud audible biphasic stridor (a different type of noisy breathing, which is a new finding). Though alarmed, we decide to replace the tube and give her some time. When the anesthesia is completely worn off, she will have another chance for a smooth emergence. In the meantime, she is transferred to the PICU. I go out to the waiting room to face her parents.

"The surgery went well, but upon awakening, Nina was clearly struggling to breathe. We decided to put the tube back in and give her some more time."

"What do you mean 'struggling,' exactly? What are you saying? How much time? Why did this happen?"

"We're not sure yet. Hopefully this is temporary."

"And what if it's not?" Lisa isn't afraid of asking tough questions. As a seasoned NICU mom, she's been down these roads before. She knows the truth in medicine. Not everything always works out.

As a seasoned NICU mom, she's been down these roads before. She knows the truth in medicine. Not everything always works out.

"Let's give it some time. Try not to worry."

We give Nina steroids to decrease inflammation. Hours later, a repeat attempt at extubation is partially successful. She still has loud, effortful breathing. I perform a bedside scope exam to figure out why. As soon as the image of her airway fills the screen, the reason is obvious. Between her two vocal cords is just a sliver of space. For a patient to breathe comfortably, their vocal cords need to open widely with each inhalation. Nina's left cord already didn't open due to her previous nerve injury as an infant. Her right side had always been able to do all the work of excursion. But now the *right* vocal cord just sits there, quivering, not opening. She is breathing, but passively, as if through a tiny straw.

Despite continued noisy — and visibly strained — breathing, Nina initially holds her own. Drinking does not go so well. She seems to have regressed considerably. She is clearly coughing and choking on water. We order a swallow evaluation for the following day, which she promptly "fails." She is only cleared to drink very thickened liquids.

We observe Nina for several more days in the hospital without an event. Things are no worse, but also no better. Finally, she is discharged home in stable condition, as per her parents' request. Her parents are extremely capable, and I know they'll return at the first sign of any trouble. This is the point at which I give Lisa my cell phone number. As always, I am praying not to hear from her. But, two days later, I receive this text …

"Hi Dr. Lando. It's me. We are bringing Nina to the Emergency Room and she's not doing well."

During the next week, we re-admit Nina, restart steroids, and just wait. We keep her in a safe environment with oxygen monitoring while asleep. Despite our optimistic expectations, Nina does not improve with time. She becomes quiet, almost withdrawn. Her bright eyes look sullen. She doesn't want to hop around on one foot, even though I know she can. She doesn't want to do much of anything, clearly conserving all her energy for breathing.

After almost two weeks of this, her father, Ron, decides, "I can't watch her like this anymore. Please do whatever you can to make her comfortable again."

Lisa nods.

"Yes, whatever she needs."

The following day, I bring Nina back to the operating room to open her neck again. This time, it's to place a plastic tube in the center of it.

TIME-OUT

This is a 2.5-year-old female who is returning to the operating room for placement of a tracheostomy after experiencing persistent respiratory distress and right vocal-cord dysfunction of unknown etiology following a surgery on her already-paralyzed left vocal-cord nerve two weeks ago.

This is not a surgery I ever wanted to do. Not on her, sweet Nini.

In character, Lisa and Ron nimbly adjust to the shock of bringing Nina home with a trach. Their love for her immediately trumps any trepidation related to her care. I, on the other hand, am wracked with guilt. For weeks, I have nightmares in which I have performed a wrong-side operation (I had not). I repeatedly wake up in a cold sweat, struggling to envision her *left* pink neck scar.

At first, I continue to hold out hope for spontaneous recovery.

At first, I continue to hold out hope for spontaneous recovery.

Why not? Nerves recover from "stunned" injuries all the time.

Why not her? Why not now? Especially since there is no clear mechanism of injury at all.

Instead of improvement, a series of other perplexing events occur.

On more than one occasion, Nina's oxygen levels drop inexplicably even though her tracheostomy tube is wide open. She has episodes of bradycardia (slowed heart rate). There are several middle-of-the-night ER visits with spontaneous resolution of symptoms just as mysteriously as they appeared.

I am convinced there is a key to it all. A neurological issue must have been missed! Something associated with her ultra-preemie brain? Some underlying cause that has always been there but is now just manifesting? I order a brain MRI and an EEG, and I obtain a neurology evaluation ... Nothing.

There is a mechanism of testing the electrical signal of a nerve called electromyography (EMG). In bigger, more accessible nerves, this can easily be performed by a neurologist in the office. For young children, to test the nerves to the voice box, it needs to be performed under anesthesia. Maybe *this* can shed more light on the case.

TIME-OUT

This is a (now) 3-year-old female with a known left vocal-cord paralysis, tracheostomy, and inability to open her right vocal cord after a surgical intervention. She is here today for an airway re-evaluation and laryngeal EMG to test the electrical signal to her right vocal cord. The neurophysiologist is present to interpret the results of nerve monitoring.

There is a distinct buzz in the air when Nina is brought to the OR. Everyone on staff knows her story. They know how upset I am and how much I am hoping for clarity from these results (for peace of mind, at the very least).

The exposure of Nina's airway proceeds uneventfully. The small joints of her larynx are normal and mobile, ruling out another possible explanation of joint fixation (immovable joints). As expected, the proper placement of the electrodes in that small space is difficult and time-consuming. When we finally hear that beautiful beeping sound — the sound of a nerve firing — emanating from the right-sided electrode, the entire room applauds. If the signal is intact, the nerve is electrically intact. And if the nerve is intact, there is still hope … Isn't there?

Over the next months, here and there are signs of progress, like when she finally stops needing those damned thickened feeds and just starts swallowing normally again.

In young children, testing the nerves that control the voice box must be performed under anesthesia. Maybe this test can shed more light on the case.

Will her right cord start moving again? Will the nerve awaken from its slumber?

I keep checking.

So far, it has not.

DEBRIEF

"Sometimes you can do everything right and things may still go wrong."

That is one of the hardest lessons to learn and I still grapple with it to this day. No surgeon wants to believe it and I guarantee no parent ever wants to hear it either.

All surgeries have risks. Heck, everything we do in life does. "Operative risk" is a complex term that includes many patient-related factors, surgical factors, and system-related factors. The problem is that it also includes random and unpredictable things, too.

As surgeons, we are charged with counseling parents on the risks of surgery so they can make proxy decisions for their children. In practicality, obtaining parental "informed consent" while taking care not to incapacitate them with fear is a tricky balance. If before every tonsillectomy, I warn the parent that the risk of surgery includes their child bleeding to death or never waking up, I am sure to reduce them to a puddle of tears, forever holding the pen in their hand and mired by indecision.

When things do go wrong, how do you manage? Especially when there are no answers, when there is never a "Eureka" moment? When there is nothing that you could have done differently to prevent it from happening again … except to never have done it at all?

There are choices for Nina, regarding decannulation (getting the tracheostomy tube out). Most require the creation of space, to pry open the vocal cords away from each other enough that she can breathe through the space between them. But with the creation of space — either by wedging the cricoid cartilage open with a graft or by cutting out a wedge with a laser — there are risks too. First off, there is the risk of degradation of her voice, the very thing we started this whole journey to improve. Secondly, as she has demonstrated time and again, she may begin to aspirate into her lungs … even though this risk is lower in older children and even though in the past, Nina has eventually recovered her normal swallowing ability.

Lisa always says, "If anyone is going to be one in a million, it's my Nini."

Of course, Nina's voice outcome is excellent. Yet, despite her generous hugs, most of the time she absolutely refuses to speak to me in the office. For proof of her conversational fluency, Lisa texts me adorable video clips from home in which Nina is yapping away, pretending to be "Dr. Yando" (me) while examining her dolls with her pink and purple Doc McStuffins otoscope.

Of the countless families I have cared for, Nina's family is unique. They maintain that rare perspective of the proverbial glass being half full. This does not preclude being upset or disappointed by reality. This mentality does not require that things be perfect or even easy. Still, their perspective is something I cherish about them. They just have one clear goal: for their daughter to be happy … and she is. They just want her to live a full life … and she absolutely does. Nina goes to school and plays with her friends. She even swims with her tracheostomy capped and her cute head bobbing above the water.

As a surgeon, I so badly want to solve her problem myself — to right what went wrong, even if there is no fault. But it's not a matter of what I want for her. I have presented options and various highly competent referrals. For now, her adoring, well-informed parents have firmly decided to give her time to grow. It is unlikely to solve her problem of space, but one day soon, I believe smart, spunky Nini will tell us exactly what *she* wants. And we'll be listening.

At Home

At my low points, I strive to remind myself that the reason the stakes always feel so high in this profession is because they are. I'm not a plumber, though I may unclog the ear "pipes." I'm not an electrician, though in some cases I am "reconnecting the power." I'm not a mechanic, though I may try to fix things.

The reason the stakes always feel so high in this profession is because they are.

Unlike most other professions, if the outcome is bad during *my* workday, it's a person's life and health at stake. And to add to it, in pediatric surgery, it's a *child's* life. I know that in surgery there is no room for human error. The only problem is that these surgeries are being performed by humans (who are imperfect) on people whose bodies may be flawed, too. This level of stress can be overwhelming at times. It leads to high rates of marital distress, divorce, mental anguish, and physician "burn-out." It is psychologically taxing and all-consuming.

Nina's case was never totally gone from my mind. After initial hesitation, I began to perform that same surgical procedure many more times. Each time, the result has been a wonderful improvement of the voice, as expected. Still, I continued to search under every stone, presenting Nina's case informally to experts on several occasions (even when it made me uncomfortable to do so, maybe *especially* then).

The November before publishing this book, I attended a highly specialized surgical conference entitled "International Workshop on Unilateral and Bilateral Laryngeal Reinnervation." It is taught by the guru of laryngeal nerve surgery, Dr. Jean-Paul Marie. The course is set in a modern glass building called the Medical Training Center in the town of Rouen, Normandy. It is not an easy place to reach.

Despite the long international schlep, I was pumped for this fascinating seminar with ENT surgeons gathered from all over the world, including England, Holland, Turkey, Saudi Arabia, Australia, and elsewhere. I attended the lectures, participated in the gross anatomy dissection, and took notes on the surgical tips and tricks. I even dissected a raw chicken thigh and performed neurorrhaphy (the surgical suturing of a divided nerve) under a microscope. I also went out to dinner with my new colleagues and even shopped a bit along the city's charming cobblestone streets.

In truth, I flew all the way to France searching for answers.

I wanted to ask Dr. Marie one specific question, in person.

Delayed by the pandemic, I had waited four years for this moment.

When the time seemed right, I raised my hand.

I relayed Nina's entire story. I paused to let the details sink in.

"Dr. Marie, why do you think this happened?"

All eyes fixed on him as my question hung boldly in the air.

He replied simply with his charming French accent.

"To tell you the truth, Dr. Lando, I just don't know."

A WORD ABOUT THE NEXT SURGICAL CASE

Needless to say, not every part of our job as surgeons is so serious. Some of the scenarios we face in our hospital are downright outrageous. Even when it's the middle of the night, you have to find the humor in them. If you don't grab onto a buoy in the shit storm, you're gonna burn out fast.

If I can get a good belly laugh at least once a month, I'm set for a while. Bonus points for me if I can make someone around me crack up too.

So, readers, if you're still with me, here's one for a bit of Shakespearean comic relief. Then, we can all return to my heart-thumping stories of life and death.

I give you "The Cocaine Condom."

CHAPTER 7

THE COCAINE CONDOM

As I've mentioned, I am an ENT surgeon who special-
izes in caring for children. So, I should *not* be dealing with condoms
… or cocaine … let alone both … at the same time … at 2:00 a.m.
… inside the body of a heavily tatted 44-year-old prisoner.

But here I am anyway …

My medical practice has worked out a system whereby, on
the weekends and nights on call, we attendings (pediatric ENTs)
supervise ENT consults for the entire medical center. This is not
the case in many other major hospitals, where the line between
pediatrics and the adult world is drawn firmly in the sand. The
advantage of this arrangement is fewer days a month of sleep disruption, but the disadvantage is a greater intensity and breadth of
our responsibilities when we are "on call." This agreement requires
us to step out of our subspecialty comfort zone, which for me means
dealing with adult problems.

Because our hospital is situated on the same property as
a county jail, we can get some rough characters coming through
the ER doors. One of the issues we — as ENT surgeons, both
pediatric and adult — routinely deal with is foreign-body ingestions

and inhalations. Simply put, that means fishing out various objects from places they don't belong, like the esophagus or, more treacherously, the airway. Lucky for us, for the lower-down problems (and there are *MANY*) get punted to the GI doctors and general surgeons.

On this particularly auspicious night, one burly inmate had a special jailhouse visitor. During their brief encounter, a grayish black package the size of a Gherkin pickle was transferred from visitor to prisoner. It is unclear to me if the contents of this exchange were intended for personal use or for wider distribution. Needless to say, in an attempt to smuggle it "inside," the prisoner swallowed the sachet in one giant gulp. His plan was to naturally release the bundle at a later, less conspicuous time, and retrieve its contents intact. The only problem was that it got stuck. Like … really stuck.

Time-Out

This is a 38-year-old male inmate who was brought into the ER by ambulance in severe distress with inability to swallow his own saliva and with searing chest pain. He is here for removal of an esophageal foreign body, suspected to be a parcel of drugs.

When a big wad of material gets jammed in the esophagus, the esophagus contracts against it. This involuntary wave-like movement of the muscles in the GI tract is called peristalsis. When the object is not successfully expelled, the muscles go into spasm. This experience feels as excruciating as a heart attack. That is why this 6'4 muscular mountain of a man with neck-to-arm-sleeve tattoos was writhing in pain when I stumbled into the adult side of the hospital, bleary-eyed, but ready to rock n' roll.

The gentleman's pre-op CT scan of the chest revealed, "A non-metallic multilayered object lodged in the upper segment of the esophagus."

This proximal location should be easily accessible with our usual rigid metal equipment (cervical esophagoscope), or so I thought. My resident, Sara, and I set up all the standard telescopes and grasping forceps in OR 10. Soon after, the loopy patient is wheeled into the room, handcuffed to the side rail and accompanied by his prison guard. John (as we'll call him) is finally chillaxing from the sedating effects of his premedication. He is no longer thrashing about, crying for his mom or "the fucking bastard" who swore he could swallow and poop the drugs right out. While we wrestle the patient onto the OR table, the guard parks himself on a free stool and immediately nods off to sleep.

SURGERY START TIME — 1:45 A.M.

The patient is now fully anesthetized and intubated, which definitely calms down the tone of the operating room. During induction of anesthesia, the esophageal sphincters (upper and lower) also relax due to the effects of the medications as well as loss of control over the swallowing reflex. This often loosens jammed objects as the muscle stops tightly spasming against them, but not always.

As per protocol, I allow the on-call resident "first crack" at removing the special package. She sits down, places the tooth guard and carefully passes the rigid esophagoscope down the back wall of his pharynx (throat). She suctions all the pooled secretions and then introduces the straight zero-degree telescope to visualize the target. We note that the object is lodged a bit lower down than expected from the imaging. On closer inspection, all we can see is a full screen of grey-black mound. What we absolutely can't identify is an edge or anything whatsoever to grab onto. For the next thirty minutes, I remain convinced that all we need to do is rotate the thing around just so. Then, we can locate where it is tied, engage the knot, and voila! Get in, get out, then get back home to my comfy bed before sunrise.

Four-five minutes later, despite the freezing temperature of the room, my resident starts to sweat. Around her light-blue mask, her skin is visibly flushed. Her brow is deeply knitted in frustration. Unwilling to concede easily, she keeps unusually quiet, clearly hoping I won't notice her lack of progress. As a rule, residents don't willingly relinquish these cases to their attending, especially not the senior trainees. Yet, after another half an hour of entirely futile effort, Sara stands up in exacerbation and moves aside without any encouragement necessary.

Four-five minutes later, despite the freezing temperature of the room, my resident starts to sweat.

"Over to you, Boss!"

She storms off to return several missed texts, in an emotional state I can only describe with the Yiddish term "farklempt," meaning choked up or emotionally squeezed.

When I take over, I intend to wow everyone as the seasoned pro. Twist, grasp, yank.

C'mon, Tali, show them how it's done.

But the thing is *so* wedged, I can't get around it at all. The drug sack is double layered in some type of thick rubber condom. It is such a slippery little sucker. Whenever I get a tenuous hold of the side, it flips around again. After a few more failed attempts, I start cursing ... like *a lot.*

SHIT. FUCK. BLEEP BLEEP ...

It only gets worse from there. At least another hour goes by, during which time I use every grasping instrument I can find, in an attempt to get a purchase. It is so smooth and tight.

"Ok, this is clearly not working."

In a change of tactic, I switch over to vascular balloons. If I can snake a balloon past it, then I might be able to engage and pull back. Maybe that will loosen the damn thing and drag it more proximal. Multiple balloon inflations later and ...

No such luck!

Conversely, there is also the "the push technique." This involves pushing the object deeper into the stomach, where there is more room to maneuver the instruments. Then, the GI folks can remove it. This is a reasonable option, in theory, but there are no gastroenterologists awake to take over even if I am successful. Anyway, when I attempt to nudge the package forward, the resistance is too high. I'm convinced this method will perforate the esophagus. Then, my already *big* problem is sure to become a *giant* one.

It is 3:30 a.m. when I finally wake up the GI attending. He advises, "Try glucagon. It further relaxes the smooth muscle of the esophagus and the lower esophageal sphincter. You can also try calcium channel blockers." The sleepy voice on the line does not offer to come assist. He assuredly does not suggest I call back if I need help using endoscopic GI instruments (that are clearly out of my wheelhouse).

So, back on the frontline, we administer the recommended medications and wait … No dice. The grey gherkin does not budge.

The last (and, by far, least-appealing) option is a thoracotomy (opening the chest) to perform a surgical esophagectomy (cutting into the esophagus). This would require a general or thoracic surgeon, also possibly asleep at home, although often lurking around somewhere in the hospital at all hours. It's an invasive surgery that would require first waking the patient from anesthesia, obtaining informed consent, and arranging a separate surgical intervention. It could take hours and has serious risks and recovery time.

When it comes down to it, I have to make a call, and I do. This is my job.

I know the last option is to puncture the outer bag. It is the very thing I have been avoiding all this time. I decide that, if done properly, it is the lesser of all the evils. With careful conviction, I make a tiny nick in the outer condom. Underneath, I can see the edge of a clear plastic knot. If I can just grab it …

Slowly, but surely, my forceps grasp and displace the bag upward a few millimeters. Then, I wiggle and jiggle and finally free it up through the esophageal inlet and out of the mouth.

Success, Girrrl!!!

Well, mostly. Before I pass the evidence to the police, I notice a miniscule hole in the *inner* plastic double baggie.

I nudge awake the knackered, snoring, uniformed man with the handcuffs, eager to dispose of the contraband.

"Here you go sir. One big 'ole bag of drugs. Now *this* is why I prefer dealing with kiddos."

Soon after, I hear the pitch of the heart rate intensify and the cycled blood pressure reading jumps super high. I open the patient's eyelids, and his pupils are enormously dilated.

Crap sandwich!

My own pulse rate rises to match the convict's. I'm crossing my fingers behind me as I wait for his vitals to level off.

During the next few minutes, we all stare transfixed at the monitor until the patient mercifully stabilizes. Lucky for me, his autonomic nervous system is already very tolerant of large doses of heavy drugs.

For the following half an hour, the patient remains not exactly awake but definitely high as a kite.

It is five o'clock in the morning.

At this point, we face the hot-potato, middle-of-the-night, recovery-room dance. The nurses in the post-anesthesia care unit (PACU) call "not it" by refusing to accept the patient. They are not comfortable taking care of a "jacked-up-criminal-on-coke." The medical and surgical ICUs won't take the patient because they have limited beds and declare him "not *unstable* enough to be an appropriate ICU candidate." As always, the ER always claims "no backsies" and never accepts a patient who has already left their unit. The regular floor team claim he's "*too unstable, talk to the ICU.*" So, here we are, trapped in the post-surgical limbo circle of Dante's Inferno.

After five more pleading phone calls, escalation of the issue to nursing administration, followed by high-level negotiations, we reach a settlement. The patient will continue to be observed in the operating room for an additional agreed-upon period of time to ensure his stability and manageability in the recovery room. He will then be accepted to PACU for two hours and, afterward, to the ICU overnight to manage any short-term issues with his hemodynamic status. From there, he will be expeditiously discharged back to prison.

And just like that ... one day later, the impacted prisoner leaves our institution. He's still shackled but in absolutely pristine physical condition, sober, and completely "unplugged."

DEBRIEF

Body packing is a big problem in healthcare. The endoscopic extraction of these objects is not generally favorable because rupture of package contents has dangerous consequences. The drugs are often encapsulated tightly in multilayer well-wrapped packets, which is good, but it makes them extra slippery for grasping. The typical dictum is "do not puncture the bag." Obviously, a massive quantity of hard drugs released into the bloodstream can be lethal. This should be avoided at all costs. The promise in our oath to "do no harm" stands no matter how stupidly the patient behaved. It is chiseled into the consciousness of every physician.

Fundamentally, this story is about making tough choices. In the OR, the surgeon is the pilot. Ultimately, like Maverick, you have to "call the ball." Even when it's the middle of the night — even when you can't fully predict the outcome but you know you've reached an impasse. You make the call because long-term parking in the operating room is not an option. The impact of wasting time there isn't only about money. Each extra minute you occupy that room in a major medical center may cost the life of another patient waiting for surgery in the emergency room or the intensive care unit.

So, I tell my medical students about this litmus test when they are making that big decision between surgery or other medical specialties: "There are lots of different kinds of doctors, and you can be any one of them. But there is one thing you gotta determine if you want to be a surgeon: Do you have the cojones when it comes to making the rent in the cocaine condom? If not, the operating room may not be the place for you."

AT HOME

It's been a long call-weekend. I get home around 7:00 a.m. and slink under the covers. I'm so overtired, I can't fall asleep. So, true to form, I start making lists in my head.

- Bring down the camp trunks (where are they?).
- Make yearly physical appointments for every member of the household (all overdue).
- Finish my office notes (or at least some).
- Call the plumber to fix the garbage disposal (again).
- Call the peds pulmonologist to coordinate the flexible bronchoscopy case with the sinus surgery (actually, two cases).
- Go to the supermarket because we're out of *everything* (including milk, eggs, and fruit) or ask Alex to do it (we both know he's more likely to follow through anyway).
- Buy light bulbs for the hallway and batteries for the remotes and then actually install and replace them, respectively.

- Buy satin pillowcases or hair bonnets to tame frizzy hair (not mine).

The only thing I accomplish is the last one because I'm excellent at Amazon shopping in bed. Also, I do start one patient note because my computer is already on my nightstand. I leave the other 99 delinquencies unfinished. Mercifully, I fall into a deep sleep with my cell phone on max volume — carefully positioned by my right ear, as always, during call weekends.

Ten minutes later, my phone rings. It's the transfer center who wants to connect me to the ER in a referring community hospital two hours away with a patient who was assaulted with a box cutter.

Fuck all — we're covering facial trauma this week. I forgot.

"Is the patient in acute respiratory distress?"

Once they answer "no," I'm already half back asleep.

"Yes, yes, I'll accept the transfer. Please page the ENT resident on arrival. No updates necessary."

Now for the love of G-d, let me sleep.

Another fifteen minutes pass. It's 8:00 a.m.

Always on cue, Milla pops up at the foot of my bed.

"I'm HUNGRRRY!!!!!"

"Just go downstairs and find something. Anything."

"But I want *you* to come with me."

Yawn, pleading ... and then the unavoidable parental submission.

The transition between the adrenaline-inducing and the mundane aspects of life can be tough, but I try to take it in stride. I cherish the calm parts of parenting but thrive on the sporadic heart-stopping moments of the job. If I could divide my life into equal parts, leisurely drinking my morning coffee on the porch with

Alex and endoscopically managing infant airways in the afternoon, I'd be golden. But there's a ton of shit in between. Also, it's the simultaneous nature of it all that can be the hardest part. Like, as soon as I promise Juliette ten minutes of undivided attention (for the hundredth time), that's when my phone inevitably rings for …

I cherish the calm parts of parenting but thrive on the sporadic heart-stopping moments of the job.

"I know you're not on call … *but* …"

There's also the exhaustion that makes you grumpy. Even though we're trained to jump into action in the middle of the night, that doesn't mean we really want to.

Once, when I was a single young resident in NYC, I was called in for an airway emergency in the middle of the night. I was darting across York Avenue, as a cab was running the red light through the crosswalk. I didn't have enough time to dive out of the way and was sure I'd be hit head on. Either due to good luck or divine intervention, the car screeched to a halt within an inch of my life. I was shaken, but all I could think was that no one would realize I was dead until morning. After all, no one knew I left my bed. They'd only notice when the pissed-off ER attending reported me for ignoring the damn pager.

These are the disturbing thoughts you have at 1:00 a.m. on a Saturday morning when the only other people awake are drunkenly stumbling out of clubs. Nevertheless, I know I'm blessed. I wake up every day with a clear sense of purpose. It's not always grandiose. I'm not always "saving lives" (like my kids think I am). But I *am* often making some child's life a bit better, enabling them to hear or breathe or sleep more restfully. Like everyone, some days I'm dragging (despite three cups of coffee) and others, I'm raring to go. Mostly, my days are packed with routine problems like big tonsils, ear fluid, and sinus infections. Some find that monotonous, and that's ok. For me, if I get to recharge my battery with the occasional rush of "that-was-bat-shit-craaazy," I'm still diggin' the journey.

CHAPTER 8

CYSTS, PITS, AND THE BULLFROG EFFECT

CONGENITAL NECK CYSTS are a frequent otolaryngologic problem in children. They can occur in various locations in the middle or sides of the head and neck. Their location alludes to their developmental origins. I have always been fascinated by the various manifestations of these anomalies — these vestiges from an intricate process that begins very early in embryonic life. Even more so, I love the challenge of removing these remnants when they become a problem. Each case is unique, a specific watermark of human formation gone slightly awry. Sometimes, rather than an entire mass, an opening (otherwise known as a pit or fistula) or just a small piece of misplaced cartilage remains.

The most common type of neck cyst is called a thyroglossal duct cyst. Early in gestation, our thyroid gland begins to form from a thickening at the base of the tongue called the foramen cecum. Over time, this gland migrates downward to its destination in the lower midline of the neck. During this process of descent, a tract forms, known as the thyroglossal duct. An abnormal persistence of these ductal elements leads to the formation of cysts. These cysts can lay dormant inside us like deflated balloons. Thyroglossal duct cysts often pop up during childhood (90% before the age of 10 years). Most of these patients present to my office with neck masses, often incidentally noticed by parents during bath time or when the child throws their head back in a tantrum. Other times, I first see the patient in the emergency room with a large, painful, red lump — often following a simple cold. When the cyst is badly infected, the child can have difficulty swallowing and — depending on the exact location — even problems breathing as well. That's how I met Hadley.

Time-Out

This is a five-year-old, otherwise healthy, female with an acutely infected thyroglossal duct cyst, which has not responded to two days of IV antibiotics. She is here today for drainage of the abscess cavity with a plan to send the fluid specimen for culture.

Hadley is an adorable five-year-old with a blond braided ponytail and two frilly pink bow clips. By the time I meet her, a CT scan has already revealed a large cystic midline neck mass extending into her tongue. She is uncomfortable swallowing, and her fever and white blood cell count are elevated. The initial plan is to admit her for at least 48 hours of IV antibiotics and observation to "cool down" her active infection. Typically, definitive surgical excision is delayed for four to six weeks. This allows the surrounding inflammation to resolve. If the patient does not improve, an initial incision and drainage procedure may be necessary to help calm the infection.

Surgery Start Time — 2:15 p.m.

Traditionally, in these abscess cases, the resident is given the honor of making the initial "stab incision." First, it makes their day. Second, there's virtually no way to screw it up!

Chris, my junior resident, grabs the blade with excitement.

Yellow fluid doesn't just ooze out of the wound; it erupts like "Old Faithful."

The OR peanut gallery utters various "oohs" and "aahs." Chris is giddy with delight.

Hey, there's a reason Dr. Pimple Popper has over five million followers on social media — abscess drainage is incredibly satisfying. Everyone in the room, except the one doing the popping, is always a little bit envious.

The first time I was sure my husband really loved me was when, after I came home from draining a neck abscess during my ENT residency, he had learned to ask, "So, sweetie, did you get pus?"

"Yes, yes, I did. Thanks for asking!"

After the drainage is complete, we culture and irrigate the wound. Hadley does great, starts to improve, and is discharged two days later on oral antibiotics.

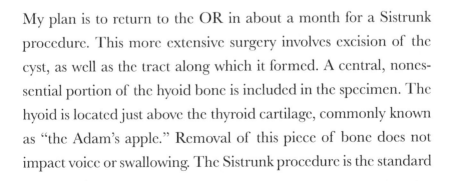

My plan is to return to the OR in about a month for a Sistrunk procedure. This more extensive surgery involves excision of the cyst, as well as the tract along which it formed. A central, nonessential portion of the hyoid bone is included in the specimen. The hyoid is located just above the thyroid cartilage, commonly known as "the Adam's apple." Removal of this piece of bone does not impact voice or swallowing. The Sistrunk procedure is the standard

technique for treating this condition, though several nuanced varia-
tions exist depending on the surgeon's preference. The main goal of
the surgery is to eliminate the problem and to prevent recurrence.

Five weeks later ...

TIME-OUT

*This is a five-year-old female who was taken to the OR last month
for I&D of an abscess. She is here today for Sistrunk Procedure with
the Koempel method. Dr. Yao will be assisting with the tongue-base
portion of the procedure.*

Typically, I do not preemptively involve Dr. Mike Yao in these cases
unless they are revisions. In this case, I knew (from prior imaging)
that the cystic elements penetrated the base of the tongue. As a head
and neck surgeon, Mike is constantly involved in cancer-related
resections of the tongue so he is an expert in this anatomy. More
than that, he is just an overall great guy, a talented surgeon, and
a pleasure to collaborate with. Rather than asking him to be on
standby as backup — which can be very disruptive to his schedule
— I planned to have him there from the start.

SURGERY START TIME — 7:45 A.M.

Overall, the case goes smoothly. As expected, there are still numerous
adhesions — sticky attachments to the surrounding tissues — from
the recent, nasty infection. This makes the dissection a bit more
challenging, but still entirely manageable.

Once skeletonized, the cyst is about a third the size it was when infected. I peel it away from the surrounding neck muscles. The central portion of the hyoid bone is identified, and I use heavy scissors to release it on either side. The lateral parts of the bone are left in place to protect the nerves that control tongue movement. On the inner surface of the hyoid, a second cyst extends deep. At that point, Mike scrubs in to assist. Together, we proceed to fully isolate the remaining portion of the problem.

Chris (back again) is instructed to place a gloved hand into the patient's mouth, purposely "breaking scrub." In this kind of procedure, you need the tactile feedback from feeling the collaborating surgeon's fingertip on the other side of the thin lining of mucosa between the mouth and neck. My still-sterile finger touches his fingertip from inside the neck wound. All these careful maneuvers are meant to prevent this problem from ever recurring.

After the entire specimen is removed from the body, it is placed on the draped Mayo stand (portable instrument stand) for further inspection. It looks like some kind of sea creature.

"It's a doozy alright."

Everyone looks over to remark on the size of "Thomas," our newly christened thyroglossal duct cyst with hyoid bone being sent to pathology.

The final step is to inspect the wound for bleeding. We release the metal retractors to ease pressure on any blood vessels that might be in spasm. A stubborn area in the upper corner of the surgical bed keeps welling with blood. We cauterize it using bipolar cautery. The bleeding recurs, but less so. We cauterize the spot again, and this time it stops completely. We place a small piece of absorbable SURGICEL dressing in the area. This material accelerates clot formation by providing a physical matrix for platelets to adhere to. Finally, we ask the anesthesiologist to perform a Valsalva maneuver — increasing pressure in the ventilatory circuit — as a final check for hemostasis.

"Bloodless! Wonderful! Looks great. Now let's close her up and make it look beautiful."

After a meticulous wound closure and a smooth emergence from anesthesia, Hadley is transported to the recovery room. I continue with the rest of my day as planned — several more cases await, each with a hungry young patient of their own, who hasn't been allowed to eat on the day of surgery. After a standard interval of observation, Hadley is transferred to her overnight room on the third floor. Approximately an hour later, Will, the senior resident, performs the routine post-op check. Hadley is asleep on her father's lap. The gauze dressing around her neck is lifted, revealing a small amount of blood-tinged drainage from the straw-like drain — exactly as expected. According to Will's note, Hadley's neck is "appropriately flat."

Forty-five minutes later, I am still operating, finishing up a nasal surgery. Chris bursts into the OR, grasping a portable screen with white knuckles.

"Dr. Lando, you *need* to look at this."

Normally respectful and measured, Chris's urgency alarms me.

According to Chris's timeline, he entered Hadley's room around thirty minutes after Will's departure. Chris also found Hadley and her father asleep in the bed. However, he was alarmed at the sound of her breathing.

"Something wasn't right. It sounded strange and gurgly."

On closer inspection, he notices that Hadley's entire neck below the jawline is tense and swollen.

"She looked like a bullfrog, so I ran to get the scope."

"This is what I found." He presses play.

I stop what I'm doing and look down at the screen. Hadley's airway is tight and distorted. Chris shows me a photo of her swollen, discolored neck.

"It's a post-op hematoma."

This abnormal collection of blood under the skin can rapidly enlarge, dangerously closing off the airway.

"Get her back down here immediately. I'll let the OR desk know it's an emergency."

"Aye, aye, Captain."

Chris scurries off, allowing me to expeditiously finish my case.

When Hadley arrives in the holding area, her neck is hyper-extended. She lies as still as a statue — never a good sign in an otherwise rambunctious child. Despite the surrounding commotion, her father remains calm, smoothing her platinum blond hair and gently kissing her forehead.

"It's ok, my love. Everything will be ok."

I pull my anesthesiologist, Dr. Julia Brothers, aside. Julia is energetic and proactive. At this point, we haven't known each other long — she's relatively new — but we've already built a solid sense of trust. I've been impressed by her skill and her natural rapport with kids. Bonus: she stocks up weekly on an array of Trader Joe's snacks and leaves them out for everyone. Even better, she secretly bought and installed iPhone chargers in all the pediatric ORs — so now I never run out of juice. In short, I already kinda love her.

"Julia, her airway sucks. We have to do a fiberoptic intubation. You can give her a touch of medication to take the edge off, but otherwise she has to be sitting up and awake."

"You sure that's the best way? She's only five. She's not going to tolerate it."

"It's the *only* way."

We need to start *now.*

After one final kiss, Hadley's father is escorted to the waiting room.

TIME-OUT (HURRIED)

This is Hadley White, a five-year-old post-op from a Sistrunk procedure earlier today who has a post-op hematoma. Her airway is compromised, and we are starting with an awake nasal fiberoptic intubation and will then proceed to evaluate the wound.

I don't need to ask for quiet this time. The room is tomb-like. Everyone's eyes are glued to the screen above as I insert the rubberized black scope through the kindergartener's nose, visualizing the swollen lining of the airway. Hadley is squirming and needs to be held down. There is no other choice. Between disordered breaths and redundant, floppy tissue, I catch a brief glimpse of the black hole below. Then, it's gone.

Get the view again and then go.

Pink, black, pink, black, pink, black …

No one exhales until the intubation tube is in position.

On my first attempt, the airway eludes me.

Get the view again and then go. Just do it.

I see the black hole fleetingly and advance.

"It's in. It's in. Ok, Julia, now, get her deep."

Once Hadley is fully anesthetized, her neck is prepped. All the carefully closed layers are re-opened. When the wound is splayed apart, we find large dark clots, which we evacuate. One of them has effectively blocked off the drain. We irrigate the cavity thoroughly. Contrary to expectations, there is no active bleeder. We fastidiously inspect every area. On first pass, we find nothing. But something caused this! We can't close up again without identifying the source. We may not be so lucky next time …

"Julia, increase the intrathoracic pressure for me."

Still nothing.

"Hydrogen peroxide irrigation, please."

I peer into the wound with my magnifying loupes.

Nothing.

"Put the patient into Trendelenburg."

Julia tilts the head of the bed downward — a maneuver that can reveal hidden bleeding vessels by increasing venous pressure.

Then I see it, a small pumper most likely feeding off the larger lingual artery.

"There! There it is. Sneaky little fucker. Cautery please."

"Finally. Got it!"

The tiny stream of red halts immediately. It never starts flowing again.

I irrigate once more. The water flows completely clear. Only then is the wound re-approximated, the drain restitched, and — finally — the dressing replaced.

Once Hadley is safely extubated, I go out to the waiting room to find her parents.

"We found the culprit vessel and took care of it. It was a small bleeder, causing a big problem. Hadley is totally ok."

Without encouragement, I lean in for a hug. This time … just as much for me as for them.

DEBRIEF

"Remember to give credit where credit is due."

There is a champion in this story, and it was definitely my junior resident Chris. Bravo to him for his dedication and quick thinking. I owe him, big time.

"Follow your gut, even if you're not completely sure what it's telling you, especially when you sense that something is wrong."

"Worst case scenario, you'll be dubbed an alarmist. Best case, you may save someone's life."

"No one will ever fault you for a second check. Most likely, they'll thank you."

"Try to spot problems early so you can fix them before they escalate. The earlier you act, the better you'll be at averting disaster."

"Even when you follow all these rules, surgery still has risks."

"We do everything in our power to minimize these risks, but we can never fully eliminate them."

At Home

That night, I do not sleep. I flip and toss until my deafening alarm marks the start of the next day.

Thoughts swirled in my head in the darkness.

She could have died. What if Chris hadn't checked on her when he did? Would her father have awoken from the noise and noticed the swelling? What if it was already too late?

There is a widely held notion that bad outcomes commonly relate to surgeon incompetence or even malicious intent. This perception is heightened by salacious stories from podcasts turned miniseries about drug-addicted surgeons with G-d complexes. Actually, most of the time, the circumstances are much more banal. The reality is that we live in a highly litigious society with a cultural tendency to assign blame. Many people view lawsuits as a way to address grievances, even when no one is in the wrong. Accordingly, in addition to the absolute dread of harming our precious patients, the fear of malpractice lawsuits looms over us surgeons like a perpetually stormy sky.

In the eyes of the public, the event of a surgical complication automatically implies that an egregious error was made. This is, most often, simply not the case. As in this situation, the surgery was done properly. To ensure the highest degree of safety, two highly trained specialists lent their joint expertise. Standard technique was adhered to, and, at completion, all areas of the wound were systematically checked for bleeding. With all these measures, it still could have been a devastating result.

I could write a lot more about the near misses, of which there are countless. I could also delve more deeply into the myriad complications that can occur despite all the best intentions. This is the less victorious side to being a surgeon. This is the dark side that can lead to depression and even suicide. Many of us who are well into our careers have circled around that shadowy place where shame and regret coexist with unintended suffering.

This is the less victorious side to being a surgeon. This is the dark side that can lead to depression and even suicide. Many of us who are well into our careers have circled around that shadowy place where shame and regret coexist with unintended suffering.

In the wise words of a beloved colleague, "Remember, if you haven't experienced complications, then you certainly have not operated enough."

On both sides of the equation — patient and doctor, illness and healing — there can be unavoidable darkness.

For now, let us return to the light.

CHAPTER 9

THE BIKE ACCIDENT

THE COVERAGE SYSTEM at a major medical center is a complex infrastructure. Most medical specialties have an in-house provider — someone physically present in the hospital, like the ENT resident or the pediatric intern. That individual is always supported by an on-call authority figure. The authority figure is often a higher-level trainee, such as a senior resident or fellow. In some cases, the in-house resident reports directly to an attending physician. An attending is a fully trained doctor who has completed all levels of medical education and training, with experience that can range from newly appointed to decades into their career. As such, during nights and weekends, there's significant reliance on the reporting-skills accuracy of first-line trainees — that is, how clearly and effectively they can communicate what they see. Over time, this verbal reporting system has been supplemented by the use of videos, audio recordings, and remote access to radiologic imaging. A key part of residency training involves learning to craft and deliver succinct, well-organized one- to two-liners, especially when waking a grumpy attending in the middle of the night:

"Hi, Dr. Lando. Sorry to bother you. I just evaluated a 13-year-old who was found down in the mountains two days ago after a bike accident. He was intubated on-site and airlifted to our medical center. He's now three days post-extubation and is presenting with an acute voice change and increased work of breathing."

At the heart of it all, though, we still rely on trust. Trust in the judgment of the "man on the ground" — whether it's an intern, resident, or physician assistant — to assess the patient and answer one essential question: "Is the patient in trouble?" Yes or no.

It's the most reductive question, but also the most critical.

In this case — with the teenage cyclist — there's a pause.

"He seems comfortable. He looks stable to me."

Still, something about the case unsettles me. A feeling I can't quite shake. An ominous sense of impending doom.

"Something isn't right. We need to take a look in the OR. I'll be there in twenty."

TIME-OUT

Kevin is a 13-year-old male who was found unconscious with unwitnessed head trauma after falling from his bike while camping in the mountains with his family. He required emergency intubation at the scene. He has now been extubated for three days and developed a voice change. He is currently experiencing acute respiratory distress and presents for airway evaluation, with endoscopic intervention as needed.

When I approach the young teenager in the holding area, I see the muscles of his neck heaving above the collar of his gown. His rough breathing is audible from the OR registration desk — five feet away. He is subdued, his gravelly voice barely a whisper.

I meet his parents, who are hovering by his side, worried and eager for his relief. Kevin doesn't have time for a lengthy explanation.

"Hello. I'm Dr. Lando, the on-call ENT attending. Something is wrong with Kevin's airway. I need to figure out what it is and fix it."

"What do you *think* his problem is?"

"I suspect it has something to do with his emergency intubation by EMS."

"Ok, Doctor … please just help him."

"I will."

SURGERY START TIME — 4:29 A.M.

"Ok, folks. Let's see what we've got."

When Dr. Mike Lew, the on-call anesthesiologist, and I begin the case, it is like all other urgent airway cases in the middle of the night on a weekend. After all, this is not our first rodeo. Mike is a weird but lovable dude — capable, hardworking, and unmistakable with his '80s-style wire-rim flip-up glasses and a fanny pack strapped over his scrub pants. He wears brown leather sandals over white gym socks year-round, regardless of the weather. He rarely knows the nurses' names (so he just randomly substitutes names like Carol or Janet). He calls all patients "she" no matter how blatantly obvious their gender. And yet, despite all his peculiar quirks, there's a deep trust between us. In the OR, we move with the ease and rhythm of a well-rehearsed dance.

Pre-oxygenate ... Check IV function ... Induce anesthesia ... Mask ventilate the patient ... Rotate the bed ... Shoulder roll ... Tooth guard ... Now, it's *my* turn ...

But this time, as soon as he pushes the milky white propofol through the IV line to relax the patient, Dr. Lew cannot ventilate him. Not at all. Kevin's jaw won't open, and his chest is not rising. As his oxygen levels tumble, Kevin begins crashing.

My mind flashes to the unthinkable — the horrific image of having to tell Kevin's parents that their perfectly healthy, athletic, and charming son is gone.

Despite the panic rising in my soul, my hand steadies as I grasp the laryngoscope, searching for that sweet spot at the junction of the tongue and epiglottis — the vallecula. I peer into the lighted hole.

Something is completely blocking his airway beneath the vocal cords.

I snatch the intubation tube from the table to my right. There is no time for methodical evaluation, not even for thought — just reflex.

When the sharp edge of the plastic tube breaks through, an audible "pop" echoes in the quiet room. In that instance, I know I'm in.

Kevin's chest begins to rise and fall. His oxygen levels and heart rate return to normal.

He is stabilized for now. But it's not sustainable.

I need to talk to his parents, and they won't like what I'm going to say.

I find Kevin's mom in the dim hallway outside. The pale fluorescent lights cast uneven blue shadows — they've been buzzing and flickering for years. His dad is farther down the hall, feverishly pacing back and forth.

"Kevin is fine for now. But something was blocking his airway."

"Something, what something?"

"I don't know exactly, but I suspect it was scar tissue. I need your consent to establish a surgical airway."

"What does that mean? What are you saying?"

"I need to make a hole in your son's neck to ensure he can breathe when I remove the intubation from above."

Kevin's dad is furious. "You want to do *what?* Cut into my son? But it was just a bike ride. He's just a regular kid. We were just camping."

"I understand. It's just not safe any other way. I'm worried his airway will close back up again if the tube dislodges accidentally. This time around could be worse. This is what we must do."

"No! Absolutely not."

Kevin's father is so distraught that he storms away, stomping and clomping his shoes on the linoleum floor. Several feet down the hall, he stops and glances back, madness flickering in his eyes.

In contrast, Kevin's mother is even-keeled. Her mauve Athleta sweatpants pair perfectly with spotless white Nike Air Force sneakers and a well-fitted black spandex top. Casual yet put-together, she carries the quiet strength of a tough high-school teacher from Staten Island. Despite her internal turmoil and streaming tears, she maintains her composure.

"Yes. Whatever it takes. Save my son. I give you permission."

She locks eyes with her husband.

"*We* give you permission."

She scribbles her signature on the consent form, and I hurry back to their precious only son.

TIME-OUT (FOR SECOND TIME TONIGHT)

Intraoperative consent was obtained from the parents to establish a surgical airway. Once the tracheostomy is placed, I'll re-examine the airway from above.

The proceeding tracheostomy surgery goes smoothly. The airway is secured. Now can I figure out what the hell is going on.

It's obvious very quickly.

Kevin is a tall teenager, despite being only 13. He was "found down" — unconscious and unresponsive on the ground. Chaos followed. His family, panicked, called 911. The wooded location made it difficult for EMTs to reach him. In the effort to save his life, the first responder placed an endotracheal tube — one that was larger than ideal for his airway. As the tube was inserted, it likely sheared off a section of the tracheal lining.

When the tube was later removed in the hospital, the exposed tissue remained raw and vulnerable. Over the next two weeks, it formed a scar band that bridged across the airway, partially obstructing it. This scarring led to Kevin's breathing difficulties and his newly altered voice.

At the time of anesthesia induction — when his throat muscles relaxed — that partial blockage became a complete one. The airway only reopened when I reintubated him, snapping the scar band apart in the process.

Now, the airway looks relatively patent (open).

Under direct visualization, I inject steroids to prevent recurrent scarring.

"I need to let the airway heal and come back in two weeks to re-check."

Kevin is transferred to the recovery room. I walk out again to find the family.

"It's done. He's going to be ok."

Mom nods, her eyes glazed and puffy. Dad jumps up from his seat but doesn't look at me.

"We did the right thing," I say.

And then the dam breaks — for both of us. It was a close call. Too close. And I'm a mother, too.

It's 5:00 a.m. The sun still hasn't risen. There's no time to go home.

I catch an Uber from the hospital to meet my husband and kids at the Delta terminal at JFK. Miraculously, I don't miss my 7:30 a.m. flight for our long-awaited beach vacation — running on two hours of sleep and a double-shot espresso I grabbed on the way.

DEBRIEF

"Never dismiss a patient's personality change (specifically a child), particularly when they become quiet or withdrawn. Chances are, they are conserving their energy for a reason."

"Collaborative, shared decision-making is an ideal. This is especially true when it comes to parents and their children."

"But if time is of the essence, be persuasive in the interest of your patient."

"Parents are scared. When something must be done, you need to be real, but firm."

"Stay alert for changes in a patient's status, symptoms, or complaints."

"Watch for these signals like an electrical storm on the beach."

"When you spot them, beware of the danger brewing."

"Even if you can't see the trouble coming, always be ready to act when it does."

"Keep honing your Spidey sense of intuition."

"Learn to gauge when a critical situation is truly deteriorating, versus when it's simply suboptimal but stable. That skill will serve you well — not just in medicine, but in life."

AT HOME

In our world, there are so many "one-offs." The crazy, unlikely scenarios that almost never happen — except they do. And we see them. That's the unsettling reality of working in a trauma hospital. It's enough to turn even the most grounded parent into a paranoid one.

It's hard not to come home wanting to wrap your kids in bubble wrap, douse them in antibiotics, and keep them safely inside this cocoon forever.

It's hard not to come home wanting to wrap your kids in bubble wrap, douse them in antibiotics, and keep them safely inside this cocoon forever.

The rational part of my brain knows the odds. I know the statistics.

Yes, I've seen a healthy seven-year-old get the flu and end up in full-blown heart and lung failure — but that's rare.

Yes, I've consulted on a varsity lacrosse player who's now paralyzed from the chest down after a simple dive off a pier with friends — but that's rare too.

And yes, I've operated on a toddler with a routine sinus infection who is now partially paralyzed on one side.

Still, the chances of these things happening are exceedingly low. I know that. I really do.

Still — Kevin. He was just a kid riding his bike. His mom probably waved goodbye, maybe even called after him, "Be careful, kiddo." And the next thing she knows, I'm opening his neck at dawn.

At the airport, my girls are bickering over neck pillows and who deserves the window seat. Part of me wants to scream, "Do you know what I just saw? Do you know what I just did?"

But now, I have a different job: to become Vacation Mom. Happy Mom. Not the freaked-out, stressed, exhausted version — they get enough of her.

I will try.

They might catch glimpses: a cloud passing over my face, the clench of my jaw when my mind drifts. I can manage my tone, even my expressions — most of the time.

My thoughts, though? I can't always control where they go.

Hours later, we arrive in paradise. I'm standing by the water, gazing at the crisp blue sea, the breeze soft against my face. Even behind my oversized black sunglasses, I squint into the blazing sun.

Then suddenly, I'm somewhere else. Back in that dim hallway. I see myself talking to his parents, saying the words I prayed I wouldn't have to say: "I did my best, but I couldn't save him."

I blink hard and open my eyes.

I'm back in the here and now.

My kids are playing in the sand, building castles. And back in New York — Kevin is okay.

With a few more days of warm air and unstructured time, I'll begin to feel like a woman on vacation with her family — not a surgeon whipping her head left and right, darting in and out of OR 2 like a frenzied jackrabbit. My entire being will start to relax — even the creases in my face will begin to soften. It will feel good.

But eventually, with enough calm and stillness, a small void will begin to open. At first, it's barely noticeable — a tiny hole. Then it becomes a crater. And soon, that crater threatens to become a vast, hollow space that could swallow me whole.

That's when I know it's time to return.

To the hectic pace.

To the parent calls.

To the sea of impatient patients in the waiting room.

To the interrupted nights (well — maybe not those).

And the thwarted plans (also not ideal).

Yes, it can feel like an unwieldy burden — doctoring these young lives, tending to their parents and their relentless worry.

At times, it is a weighty sacrifice.

But it's also the greatest privilege I know.

Later

When I see Kevin in my office a month later, he's been success-fully decannulated — his tracheostomy removed. This time, his airway has healed perfectly. He's breathing quietly, comfortably, and naturally through his nose. Tall and lanky, with a charming smile, he sits across from me, proudly showing off the pink scar on his neck.

I offer to revise the scar — to make it flatter, less conspicuous — but he politely declines.

"No need," he says. "It's my badge of honor, for what I went through."

I can't help but admire this kid's resilience — his cool, easy confidence.

He shows me a video he made, which documents his medical journey. There I am — cropped blond hair, cartoonish smile — caught mid-action in a freeze-frame.

As we chat about his recovery, I learn more about him. He's interested in digital art, animation, and theater. Ice hockey is his jam.

And I can't help thinking how much he reminds me of my oldest daughter — how similar they are. Creative. Kind. Tall for their age. Both with that innate warmth, that unmistakable twinkle in their eye.

"Wow, my daughter Juliette is exactly your age and into so many of the same things."

Can I just introduce them? What are the rules of "crossing over" in this way?

At the end of the visit, I slip Kevin's mom a small, folded note with my daughter's name and iCloud address. I leave the ball in their court. Let's just see where it rolls ...

There are professional boundaries discouraging us from crossing certain lines. These hard lines mostly exist to protect vulnerable patients, but they often protect clinicians too.

In pediatric specialties, it's much more common — and often positive — to cross some boundaries. We watch our patients grow up, mature, and come into their own. Over many visits, we become personally involved with their families. It's easy to get emotionally invested. That's why it's so difficult when patients struggle, and why it feels so rewarding when our interventions help them succeed.

> We become personally involved with their families. It's easy to get emotionally invested. That's why it's so difficult when patients struggle, and why it feels so rewarding when our interventions help them succeed.

A few months later, I wander into Juliette's room. She's leaning back, long legs dangling at the edge of her bed, FaceTiming while working on an animation app called Procreate. I hear a familiar voice chuckling softly in the background.

And I know it's him. I leave them to chat for a while.

When she hangs up, she smiles.

"Kev is so nice and easy to talk to. He just gets me. I'm so *lucky* we became friends."

This was a good line to cross.

I must bite my tongue, because as much as I agree, I know luck had absolutely nothing to do with it.

READER:
AT THIS POINT, I FEEL THE
NEED TO INTERRUPT.

I cannot in good faith move forward without an important acknowledgment. Although I am the main character in these stories, there are clear limitations to my skill set. This is not an expression of false humility. None of us is an expert in everything.

At the edge of my scope and abilities, I rely on leaders in my field, colleagues and friends. Medicine has evolved into a world of "super specialists." Even so, we all co-exist within a relatively small sphere. We attend the same medical conferences. We often overlap in the care of complex patients. But I am a storyteller. I always have been. Please understand that these other unbelievably talented people are out there, diligently working — pushing boundaries, solving seemingly impossible surgical problems. Unlike me, most don't find the time or motivation to write about it.

CHAPTER 10

HEAVEN

SOME PATIENTS CHANGE you the moment you meet them. Heaven was one of them. Without intention, I connected to her instantly. Her jokester wit, squinty eyes, raspy voice, and mischievousness drew me in. When I first met her, she was living with and being cared for by her elderly aunt, Millie. Heaven had a complicated social background. Like many of my patients, she was a former micro-preemie with neonatal abstinence syndrome — born addicted to drugs — and had endured a prolonged NICU stay. As an infant, she spent months on mechanical ventilation.

When Heaven hops into my office, she is eight years old, with a gap-toothed grin, short, tight braids, and a throaty cackle. As soon as she sits in my chair, she is up again, rummaging through my drawers, and flipping all the suction switches and light buttons on and off.

Beyond her spunk, her stridor is so loud that I can hear it from around the corner. She sounds like a broken-down leaf blower. When I ask how long it's been like that, her great-aunt shrugs, "Oh, that's just Heaven. She's always been that way."

When I probe further, asking about how she handles physical activities like gym and recess, Millie replies, "She can't really do those things without getting winded. The school knows not to let her run around too much."

My first thought is, *"Hell yeah. I can absolutely help this kid. I can definitely make her life better."*

First things first — I have to gauge the extent of her problem.

TIME-OUT

Heaven is an 8-year-old ex-micro-preemie with lifelong noisy breathing and exercise intolerance. She is here today for an airway evaluation. Any more-involved intervention will be planned for a later date.

After we induce anesthesia, I let my resident, Bardia, sit down in the chair to obtain a view of the airway. Hovering over his shoulder, I remind him, "Sweep the tongue all the way to the left ... laryngoscope tip down the right gutter ... once in the vallecula, pull up and anterior at approximately a 40-degree angle. Show me your best view."

SURGERY START TIME — 7:31 A.M.

Using the zero-degree telescope, Bardia exposes the airway. The image materializing on the screen is exactly what I am expecting. Heaven has an abnormally narrowed airway beneath the vocal cords at a level called the subglottis. This area is most prone to damage from prolonged periods of intubation in the neonatal period. We grade the severity of these circumferential scars on a scale of 1-4, with 4 being the worst (no breathing hole). Heaven's grade is a 2-3, which is bad enough to have a major impact on her quality of life, but relatively favorable for repair. Fixing a damaged airway is no small task. Its technical term is "laryngotracheal reconstruction" or "LTR" in shorthand. It requires opening the neck, harvesting a piece of cartilage from the rib, intricately carving that piece to fill the gap, and then securing the graft in place. It's what we pediatric otolaryngologists are trained for in fellowship, following five years of residency and after four years of medical school before that. In my subspecialty, comfort with airway reconstruction is what distinguishes the "men (women) from the boys (girls)."

Fixing a damaged airway is no small task.

Conceptually, an LTR is straightforward — at least in terms of operative steps. After the main surgery, there are always at least two planned return trips to the OR: one for suprastomal stent removal and another for re-evaluation and possible balloon dilation. That's the predictable part. Arguably more important than the technical aspects of the primary procedure is the finesse involved. This requires experience. It manifests in the multitude of decisions made intraoperatively during the initial surgery and in the subsequent management afterward. Beyond skill and experience, there are uncontrollable variables. In airway surgery, we strive to repel the enemy forces of scarring, inflammation, and infection. We give culture-directed antibiotics (targeted at any bacteria we identify), reflux medications, and inhaled steroids, when appropriate. We involve other specialties, GI and Pulmonology, all to maximize the likelihood of success.

And despite all this collaborative effort and careful technique, sometimes children just do not heal properly.

The initial surgery on Heaven goes well. We open her neck, meticulously exposing the airway. We cut through the old scar under endoscopic visualization. We harvest the rib cartilage. Then, we fashion the anterior (front) and posterior (back) grafts to fit snugly into the structural gaps. An intraluminal (inside the airway) silastic stent is placed to support the new grafts above what was meant to be a temporary tracheostomy. Now, it is up to Heaven's tissues to heal.

As planned, we return to the OR two weeks later to remove the stent. On evaluation, the cartilage grafts appear to be properly mucosalizing — forming a healthy lining.

And despite all my best intentions, Heaven was one of those children.

It's not until the third — and ostensibly final — step, the six-week follow-up, that trouble comes knocking. Rather than revealing a nice, safe, cylindrical airway, we discover that her airway is scarring down.

As the prospects for Heaven's quick and successful recovery fade, so does the consistent appearance of her aunt Millie. At first, she stops visiting regularly. After that, she appears infrequently. Then, she stops coming altogether. We're left not only managing Heaven's airway, but also her physical safety. I want her close to the hospital — close enough to act quickly if something goes wrong. Sadly, there are no immediate family options available. We settle upon an interim plan: Heaven will stay at a nearby specialized children's facility. Within days there, the nurses rally around her, becoming temporary surrogate mothers. Still, I'm riddled with guilt over her displacement — uprooted from the only home she has ever had.

Beyond my concern with her health, I become emotionally involved in her wellbeing — too much so. Every night, as I drive home past the public elementary school on my block, I think about fostering Heaven. I rehearse the pitch to my husband a hundred times in my head. My heart wants to offer, but my brain reminds me it's impossible. At the time, I have my own three adolescent children at home, already in the hands of a caregiver while my husband and I are at work. We don't have any close family nearby. And, also, no one is even asking me. I would have to offer.

On a positive note, as Heaven's medical course stretches on, her once-absentee mother, Janelle, becomes re-involved. She starts by visiting Heaven at the rehab center. Soon, she is coming to all her medical appointments. Eventually, she even secures a steady job in retail and begins working to establish a stable home.

Unsure how deeply to insert myself into Heaven's life, I know there is one thing I can always do for Heaven. At the start of each operative case — and there are several — I am the one to connect the anesthesia circuit to her tracheostomy tube, hold her hands, look straight into her eyes, and say, "I am right here with you. Nothing will hurt you. Look at me. Relax. Breathe. Everything will be ok."

In the course of this difficult time, Heaven lost the ability to speak. She could mouth words, but she wasn't moving enough air to vibrate her vocal cords so she couldn't produce enough sound to be heard. She was already behind academically and unable to read and write. Rather than becoming despondent as I had expected, she thrived. She loved the attention of all the adoring staff in the facility. She enjoyed being the favored celebrity patient. In a world of chronically ill and neurologically damaged children, she was the queen of the castle.

In the course of this difficult time, Heaven lost the ability to speak.

As weeks turned into months — and after multiple endoscopic salvage attempts — it became clear that Heaven needed a formal revision surgery. This was her only real chance at a normal life: to breathe without a tube in her neck and return to the care of family. With the help of an expert colleague, I arranged for her to be transferred out of state to a highly specialized, high-volume airway program. Then I flew out to be there with her.

With mom's express permission, as was our ritual, I held her hands as she drifted off to anesthetic sleep.

"I am right here with you. Nothing will hurt you. Look at me. Relax. Breathe. Everything will be ok."

SURGERY START TIME (FOR REVISION AIRWAY RECONSTRUCTION) — 7:29 A.M.

I remain in the operating room for her surgery, this time as a supportive onlooker, not as her surgeon. During the case, on multiple occasions I hear the cursed phrases, "so much hardened tissue," "so much bloody scar."

As usual, she recovers easily and happily. But even with inarguably the highest level of expertise, her airway still doesn't heal properly. Days turn into weeks. More endoscopic salvage procedures are attempted. Yet despite everything, the airway stenosis — the unexplained recurrence of narrowing — persists.

At this point, Heaven has been through a lot. The decision is finally made to pause further interventions — to let her convalesce back in New York, with plans to return at a later, as-yet-unspecified date to try again.

After weeks of intensive tracheostomy-care training — including how to replace the tube in an emergency — Heaven is discharged into the care of her birth mother, to the home Janelle had worked so hard to establish.

At this point, Heaven is what we call "completely trach dependent," meaning if the tracheostomy tube is not open and unobstructed, she cannot breathe at all.

With Heaven returned physically to her family, I returned mentally to all my other patients.

Four weeks later, on a nondescript Friday afternoon, Heaven's mother calls my cell. I'm in clinic, too busy to answer at first. But when she calls again — and then again — my stomach drops. I pick up the phone ...

"She's dead."

"Who's dead?"

"Heaven. Heaven is dead. She just died."

"Slow down ... How? What do you mean? What happened? Tell me exactly."

"I was out. She was home. She was joking, laughing ... eating, just being Heaven, fooling around. Then she choked, grabbed her throat ... the tube seemed ... blocked. The babysitter couldn't help. She didn't know how to get a new trach in. By the time I got there, they had called EMS … but it was too late. They came but … but she was already gone. She's … gone."

The people around me defocused, their voices turned fuzzy like a radio station with poor reception.

How could she be gone?

Where did she go?

How do we get her back?

I was supposed to fix her.

DEBRIEF

My advice for residents:

"Do not learn from me in this case."

"Do not do what I did."

I was too close, too deep, too involved. If you can protect yourself, do it — do it better than me. I could not. Not with Heaven.

I can only repeat to you the things people told me.

"Remember that you didn't create her problem."

"We still don't know why some children scar so badly and others heal despite all odds."

"This is the nature of the beast. You cannot torture yourself."

But I did.

"You can only do so much. You made it clear that she could not be left alone with someone who could not replace her trache-ostomy tube."

But did I scare Janelle enough?

Did I repeat myself again and again until I was blue in the face? … Did I scream the words, "Without an open tube, she will die!" until my voice was lost like hers?

I don't know. I can't remember. Did I?

AT HOME

When Heaven's mother called me, I was in my office near the hospital. With a waiting room full of antsy patients, I could not take a lengthy pause. I walked two doors over to Katrina's office and started to cry.

"Tali, what's wrong?"

Like Lianne, Katrina is an extraordinary colleague who has become a true friend. She is a deftly skilled and fast otologic surgeon who remains humble and compassionate. Whether on call or not, she is always available when a child requires her specialized help. Like me, she has daughters and a spouse who both infuriates and supports her (don't we all?). She may be irritated with my constant requests to review a case, CT scan, or audiogram (hearing test), but if she is, she never lets on.

That terrible day, she listens. She hugs me.

"It's gonna be ok."

Partially revived, I return to the sea of patients with gigantic tonsils and murky middle ear fluid.

In the immediate aftermath of Heaven's death, I disconnect mentally from the sadness. I hug my children too tightly and sleep in their beds at night. Then, I bury my head in the sand of a million other demands at work and at home. I escape my sorrow through the unstoppable train of other responsibilities.

But *she* could not escape. *She* had nowhere to go.

Heaven's mom texts me that she can't live without her.

> *Yes, you can. You have to.*
> *For Heaven, for her memory.*

She texts me to say that they can't afford the funeral. So, I raise the money, partially from myself and partially from other generous donors around the hospital. I am brazen in my GoFundMe appeal, reaching out to any fellow doctor or nurse who is comfortable contributing.

She was my responsibility.

It was something to do because I couldn't bring Heaven back.

Then, one morning, I block my schedule, drive several hours up the Taconic to a small church, and work up the courage to walk inside alone.

Heads whip around as I enter. I stand out. Seated up front sits Janelle, dressed in all black.

As I approach, I kneel and then break down. I whisper in her ear the thing I didn't get to say before: "I'm so, so, so very sorry."

And rather than displace their anguish onto me, instead they call me up to the front of the church to honor Heaven. And this is what I said:

Just like with our children, doctors aren't supposed to admit they have favorites, but we do.

Heaven was one of mine. And she knew it.

Her laugh was infectious, but my favorite thing about her was her buoyant personality and unflinching resilience.

Even when things got hard, even when she could not communicate, she lit up the room.

Looking around here today, seeing nurses and therapists and caregivers and so many family members coming together in her memory is a testament to the impact she had on this world in her less than a decade of life ... Her contagious smile ... Her playful mischievousness ... Her lively strength of spirit ... It touched us all ... Our own gift of Heaven ... I promise I will never forget her.

CHAPTER 11

UNSTOPPABLE BLEEDING

ONE UNIVERSALLY ACCEPTED principle in medicine is this: you've got to love the "bread and butter" routine problems of your specialty. Some days, when I am drowning in patients, the word "love" feels like a bit of a stretch. Still, a positive attitude is essential. In pediatric otolaryngology, the "bread and butter" includes disturbed sleep, recurrent infections of the ears, nose, sinuses, and throat, chronic congestion, tonsillitis, and hearing loss. These symptoms are routine to me — but to the parents, they feel calamitous. At night, they watch in terror as their child stops breathing, struggling to inhale against a closed system. The long, frightening pauses are followed by strange gurgling noises and abrupt awakenings. Parents come into my office clutching their phones, eager to show videos of their child in contorted positions, breathing irregularly and laboriously.

"My child is gasping for air."

"I stay up all night watching them."

"How can I be sure they'll start breathing again?"

"Can they just die in their sleep?"

This phenomenon — obstructive sleep apnea — has serious repercussions, not just on parents' sanity, but on a child's behavior, emotions, and school performance. The good news? In most cases, it's easily fixable. Easy, at least, from my perspective. The most common solution is a procedure called an adenotonsillectomy, something otolaryngologists learn to perform in their very first year of surgical training. A typical tonsillectomy takes anywhere from 5 to 20 minutes, depending on the child's age, the surgeon's experience, and how often the tissue has been infected in the past.

Realistically, even the most straightforward surgery carries risk. It's not something most people like to think about — and for parents, it can be especially hard to process. For surgeons, though, it's an unavoidable occupational hazard. Postoperative bleeding is one of the most common risks across all surgical procedures. In the head and neck, the risk is amplified by the region's rich blood supply. The tonsils alone receive blood from five separate branches of a major blood vessel named the external carotid artery. That's why post-tonsillectomy hemorrhage can be so dramatic. When this small surgical site springs a leak, the result can be gorier than a horror movie.

Tonsillectomies are among the most common childhood surgeries — performed an estimated 300,000 to 500,000 times a year in the U.S. in children under 15. Most of these procedures are done on otherwise healthy kids. But where I work, the averages aren't average. We're a tertiary referral center, which means we care for the children who other practices aren't equipped to handle. These high-risk, often complex patients include kids with bleeding disorders, neuromuscular disorders, obesity, severe or multilevel airway obstruction, and a wide range of syndromes.

The risk of bleeding varies widely depending on age and other factors, and it tends to occur in two key time frames: primary (immediate, arterial) and secondary (delayed, venous) hemorrhage. Fortunately, in ideal conditions, the bleeding rate is low. The problem is, we cover not only our own patients but those of a dozen colleagues — plus countless transfers from other surgeons in the region who instruct their patients, "Just go to the nearest major hospital if there's an issue." As a result, this supposedly rare complication becomes a regular part of our on-call reality.

One of my mentors — using his disarming British accent — likes to share the "Rule of 5s" when talking to parents in the recovery room after a tonsillectomy. While not perfectly precise, it gives families a helpful ballpark of what to expect.

- ♦ 1 in 50 bleeds
- ♦ 1 in 500 bleeds badly enough to go back to the OR
- ♦ 1 in 5,000 gets transfused

And if they come back into the Emergency Department (ED)[4] and he is on call, he tells them, "Bad luck — you have the 500th kid. Let's hope they don't hit the 5,000 mark!"

It's late Saturday night when Jane arrives in our ED. She is clutching a pink bucket filled with her own blood. She is three days shy of

---

4. ED and ER are the same thing, but because the emergency department is far more than just a "room," many medical professionals prefer to refer to it more accurately as the emergency department (ED).

her 10th birthday. Pale and frightened but still alert, her piercing emerald-green eyes scan the room. Beside her, Rebecca — her mother — sits tense and exhausted, unraveling by the minute. Jane spits up bright-red blood in fits and spurts. The ED team mobilizes quickly. Within minutes, two wide-bore IV lines are in place. Vials of blood are whisked off to the lab to gauge how much she's already lost — every test marked STAT. As soon as her results hit the system, two units of O-negative blood are hung.

Few things spike your adrenaline like racing to the hospital to stop an active tonsil bleed in a child who's already lost a quarter of their blood volume … and counting.

"I'm on my way."

I arrive within 20 minutes of receiving a text picture of the "murder" scene from Usman. As I scan the lab results and vitals and absorb the gravity of what I see — Jane's blood-soaked pink Alo sweatshirt, her extreme pallor, and her tachycardia —I activate a level-one trauma. Level-one trauma signals a life-or-death emergency. It is typically reserved for near-fatal gunshot wounds, clear signs of shock, or devastating neurological injuries. It is used in crucial situations where every second counts. In cases like this, it can feel excessive — but nothing mobilizes the system faster. And in my hospital — like most — that designation is what jolts the necessary OR machinery into action.

As we gather Jane's paperwork from the nurse, the bleeding suddenly surges. She begins coughing up cups of blood at a time. The clot — the "finger on the dam" — must have dislodged, and an arterial vessel is now actively pumping. Jane is choking and starting to panic. We need to secure the airway down here. There's no time to get her to the more controlled environment of the OR.

The ER doc pushes medication as I scoot behind the head of the bed.

Jane's disoriented mom is pushed behind the curtain as we begin working.

I insert the intubation blade past her tongue, but my view of the airway is obscured by a river of red.

"Suction, on maximum high."

The pulse oximeter begins its threatening decline.

I can intermittently visualize the laryngeal inlet like the black asphalt road in a blizzard.

Focusing intensely, I catch fleeting glimpses of the V of the vocal cords and the dark hole between them.

I don't look up.

Hand outstretched, I demand:

"5.0 cuffed ETT, right hand."

To my relief, the tube slips into place. I inflate the cuff, sealing off the downpour of blood and protecting the lungs below. The bleeding hasn't stopped, but the first and most important goal is achieved: the airway is secured. We suction out the clots she's already aspirated. It's a lot — but once we're done, her oxygen saturation climbs back to an acceptable level.

"Let's roll ... NOW!"

Instinctively, Usman hops on the stretcher as I hand him a tight ball of white gauze on a long metal clamp.

"Try to identify the site of the problem."

I'm impressed by his skill as he scissors open her mouth. He's only a second-year resident, but his calm demeanor reflects a maturity beyond his training.

"I think it's the left lower pole."

He reaches in, applying steady pressure.

"I think I got it."

"Excellent job. So do I."

We both nod as the crimson tide finally begins to recede.

I hurriedly push the stretcher down the hallway between the pediatric emergency room and the main OR. There's no time to wait for permission to come up — and definitely no time to wait for transport. An ER nurse comes with us to "bag," rhythmically filling Jane's lungs with oxygen. Despite his awkward position, Usman stays completely still, maintaining his grip on the airway. We reach OR 11 six minutes later. The anesthesia and surgical teams are ready and waiting.

TIME-OUT

This is a healthy nine-year-old female with an active post-tonsillectomy bleed, approximately three days out from a total tonsillectomy performed by an unaffiliated surgeon at an outside surgery center. Her hemoglobin upon arrival is 6.8, hematocrit 19.4 (normal should be approximately 13/39). She was intubated urgently in the ED with a 5.0 cuffed ETT. The second unit of blood is running and four more units of O-negative are being sent over from the blood bank. The plan is to identify and control the bleeding. The patient will be transferred post-op to the pediatric ICU. They are aware and preparing a spot.

The on-call pediatric anesthesia team, led by our brilliant new hire — and former resident — Dr. Liana Grosinger, takes control. She places an arterial line for continuous, real-time blood pressure monitoring and administers various medications as we transfer and position Jane onto the operating table. I adjust my headlight and take my seat at the head of the bed. Though eager to assist, Usman knows I need to assess the situation first. He shifts to the side and hands me the clamp as I pry open the McIvor mouth gag. The mouth is filled with thick, scarlet-purple clots, clustered along the left side of the throat.

As tempting as it is, the goal here isn't to suction everything at once for a perfect view. It's better to move methodically — removing each clot with my non-dominant hand while cauterizing with the suction coagulator, or "bovie," in the other as I go.

SURGERY START TIME — 1:11 A.M.

After clearing the upper portion of the wound, I unroof an impressive bleeder deep at the base of the tongue — right where the palatine tonsil meets the lesser-known lingual tonsil. The suction canister fills with fresh blood.

After several rounds of delivering directed high-frequency electric current at 2,200° F, the offending vessel is finally sealed. All that remains is a patch of black char marking the battlefield.

After a few more rounds of careful inspection and repeated evaluations, I call it.

"We're done. You can wake her up. Dial the PICU and tell them we're coming."

I turn to the nearby computer to dictate the case.

Jane is emerging from anesthesia when Liana interrupts me urgently.

"Tali, you better come quick and look at this."

Blood is squirting out Jane's mouth and nose. It's not as brisk as in the ED but it's still way beyond normal.

"Shit, shit, shit. What the F?!"

Liana deepens the plane of anesthesia, and I swivel the table back around. This time, blood just keeps welling up from the depths. I can't find a specific site to cauterize.

Jane's blood pressure starts dropping. Liana starts pressors (medications to raise blood pressure).

"Ball up half a sheet of QuickClot and hand it to me on a long tonsil clamp. Quickly."

I fumble a bit until I find the sweet spot. When I apply pressure, just so, the bleeding finally stops.

"This isn't some small, isolated branch off the lingual artery. It's gotta be the main trunk. Call NeuroIR (neurointerventional radiology). She's gonna require embolization."

To my relief, Dr. Fawaz El Mufti answers his cell, and I quickly explain the situation. Despite the time, he's particularly pleasant, perhaps because I've recently operated on both of his children.

The on-call adult anesthesiologist joins Liana in resuscitating the patient. More blood is hung, along with additional clotting factors. It takes another 30 minutes before Jane is stable enough to be transferred to the interventional radiology suite. My fingertips are numb and tingling from being clenched in a fist for so long, but I don't move. My neck aches, but I don't dare uncrank it. My mouth is dry, but none of us shift. We hold our positions — just so — to keep Jane stable.

We wheel our young patient to the IR suite in lockstep. A technician helps me into a lead apron as Fawaz and his fellow gain access to the neck vasculature through an arterial line in the groin. Step one is to pinpoint the source of bleeding using fluoroscopy. The large C-arm swings into place, ready to capture a real-time image of the arterial tree. The way I'm contorted, my back has started to spasm — but I stay put.

On the first pass, everything looks normal.

"We need another view. This time, you'll need to let go so we can visualize the source."

This is scary. If I do this, I may not be able to regain control. We're not in my comfortable setting of the OR if things go sideways.

Still, I have no choice. I slowly release pressure. Predictably, blood begins to fill Jane's mouth.

"Quickly. Capture the image."

As soon as it's done, I angle myself back into the exact same position.

"Thank heaven. It stopped again."

Fawaz projects the images up on the screen.

"There it is. You see the blush? You're right. It's coming directly off the lingual artery. All that's left is a stump, like the vessel sheared right off."

Fawaz adroitly threads the catheter, snaking it from the main trunk of the large external carotid artery, then making a righthand turn into the first takeoff branch, which is the lingual. Finally, he deploys the coil.

"Now for the moment of truth."

Once again, I release pressure, this time with a little less trepidation.

Nothing bad happens. The coil holds, blocking any flow.

When I finally step into the hallway, four long hours have passed since this ordeal began. One of the nurses had already called to update the family, and Dr. El Mufti had explained the details and risks of the additional procedure.

I find Jane's parents outside the waiting room.

"She lost a lot of blood, but everything is now under control. She's gonna be fine."

"Oh, thank G-d. Thank G-d. Thank you. Thank you so much."

It's sunrise as I pull out of the parking lot, squinting to find my car — illegally parked in the circular drive, now tagged with a big green "never park here" sticker that's nearly impossible to scrape off. Twenty-five minutes later (this time I don't speed), I tiptoe into my bedroom and find Junie, our Goldendoodle, and Evie, our Cavapoo, snuggled into my side of the bed. I nudge them over. When my head hits the pillow, I hazily remember that Milla has skating lessons at nine. Hopefully, Alex will take pity on me and drop her off on the way to coaching Juliette's floor hockey game in Mamaroneck. Tomorrow, I'll call the primary surgeon to tell her what happened. It's a professional courtesy — not a chance to assign blame or complain about being up all night … tempting as that may be.

Two weeks later, on a Tuesday, I'm back on call. The main difference with weekday call is that you work the full day before and after. So, if you're up all night with an emergency, you're still expected to show up the next morning — bright-eyed and bushy-tailed. It's 11:00 p.m. Alex and I are unwinding with our nightly ritual: new episodes of *The Pitt* for suspense and old episodes of *Brooklyn Nine-Nine* for a laugh.

My phone rings, and it's Usman, who is coincidentally on call with me again.

"It's Jane again. She's back and bleeding."

"How bad?"

"So … not as bad as before and it's strange but I think it's the other side."

"Do I need to come?"

"I think so. I already called the OR and booked the case."

"Have them give IV and nebulized TXA — an antifibrinolytic that helps prevent clot breakdown. Get another set of labs. I'm heading in."

Loud groans as my feet swing over the side of the bed.

This time, we don't activate level-one. We have some time. When I meet Usman in Bay 32 of the ER, Jane is holding a new bucket, but it's nowhere near full. Her lips are caked with dried blood, but no deluge. The medication has stabilized the clot.

"Why does this keep happening?"

Rebecca has blood spatter on her crisp, white-collared blouse. She looks professional, like she is still dressed for work.

"We're gonna figure it out."

"Any family history of clotting disorders?"

"None that I'm aware of."

"OK, Usman, call hematology for a formal consult."

"Got it."

TIME-OUT (TAKE TWO)

This is a healthy nine-year-old female status post a tonsillectomy bleed on the right cauterized and then embolized two weeks ago. She again presents with bleeding ostensibly from the other side. The plan is to find the bleeder and then obtain labs for a hematologic work-up.

As Usman accurately assessed, we identify a left-sided bleeder — this time, more of an oozer. Given the time interval between the first and second episodes, it points to a lower-flow venous source rather than a high-pressure arterial one. The culprit area is broader and more diffuse than before. I place a figure-of-eight chromic suture to apply extrinsic pressure to the surrounding tissue.

The case is uneventful. This time, we admit Jane to the regular post-op floor, instead of the ICU. I make it back home just after 2:00 a.m. — not too bad. Still, I promised to handle Milla's morning routine today/tomorrow before work. That includes grumpy wakeup, unruly hair, backpack prep, and fruit smoothie. It's non-negotiable … and it's definitely gonna hurt.

Jane's initial bloodwork comes back normal — but I'm highly skeptical. A few weeks later, the full panel of specialized tests returns. The results show decreased levels of von Willebrand factor antigen and ristocetin cofactor activity — hallmarks of von Willebrand disease (VWD), an inherited bleeding disorder caused by a deficiency or dysfunction of a key clotting protein. Many girls are first diagnosed when they begin menstruating and experience unusually heavy periods, but Jane is premenstrual. Sometimes, VWD is only discovered after a patient's first surgery — or not until much later, during childbirth. Once diagnosed, preventive steps can be taken. Desmopressin is given before procedures, and clotting factors or medications like Amicar (aminocaproic acid) can be used afterward to reduce bleeding risk.

A few days later, just before discharge, I give Jane's mom my cell number. Once you've been to the altar with the same patient twice, you unofficially become responsible for them from then on. It doesn't matter who's technically on call.

Once you've been to the altar with the same patient twice, you unofficially become responsible for them from then on. It doesn't matter who's technically on call.

"I'm hoping not to hear from you."

"Trust me, so am I."

DEBRIEF

"Sometimes you think you solved it, only to realize it's something else."

"Even if you didn't create the initial problem, you're sometimes tasked with fixing it. You can curse under your breath, but in front of the patient, show grace."

"It can be frustrating cleaning up other people's messes, but some days, other people will inevitably clean up yours."

"It's ok to be off duty sometimes, but that doesn't necessarily absolve you of all responsibility. Most of us still espouse a 'you

break it, you buy it' policy. Once you get deeply involved with a patient, even if you did not perform their initial surgery, it rarely matters whose name is listed in the on-call schedule."

"Know the alternatives when the tactics at your disposal fail, because they will at some point."

"Form relationships with other specialists in the hospital and make sure to get their cell phone numbers!"

"It's essential to have intervention options outside your wheelhouse. You may need them in a pinch."

AT HOME

I've just settled onto the gym bleachers when the text comes in. Despite my best intentions to be on time, it's already the end of the first period. I've missed the last two home games thanks to unanticipated "add-on" cases tacked onto my OR days. This time, I promised my daughter I'd be present.

"I'm not on call. I'm not coming from the OR. I will definitely be there, Scar."

"It's important to me. Please make it."

"I will."

"You sure?"

"Yes, I am 100% sure."

Somehow, I still manage to get waylaid by my final few patients, whose parents had more than the average number of questions and concerns.

Before I check my phone, I try to catch Scarlett's attention. She's already on the basketball court so she doesn't notice me.

I glance down at my screen.

It's Jane's mom.

> *Dr. Lando. SHE'S BLEEDING AGAIN!!!!*

WTF? For the third time? You've got to be kidding me. This just cannot be.

> *Where are you?*

> *Already en route. We're 15 minutes out. Dr. Lando, I'm really scared.*

> *I know. It's gonna be ok. I'm coming.*

Even though she didn't register my arrival, Scarlett instantly notes my departure out of the corner of her eye. She's still in the game, so her expression doesn't overtly shift — but I see her shoulders slump, just slightly, as I slip out the exit. She doesn't look angry or even disappointed. Just … resigned.

As I travel the familiar route from the school to the hospital, my mind drifts to a Hulu special I watched recently — about Dr. Ann Burgess, the phenomenal woman who helped pioneer the field of victimology. The documentary follows her groundbreaking work in the 1970s, flying back and forth to Langley Air Force Base to assist the FBI in profiling serial killers. Her two adult sons and one daughter reflect on what it was like growing up with a mother so consumed by her work. The sons speak with pride about her accomplishments. But I couldn't take my eyes off the daughter. When she spoke about her childhood with an absentee mother, all I saw was resentment.

Back at the hospital, I find Jane tucked in the back corner of the Emergency Department. Rather than lips covered in blood, there's a red trail from her nostril to her chin. She's clearly had a recent nosebleed.

"I just sneezed twice, and it started gushing," she explains tearfully.

It's been more than five weeks since surgery, so the tonsil and adenoid beds are fully healed by now. Jane's still receiving clotting treatment, so even with von Willebrand's disease, something doesn't add up.

There's a problem-solving principle known as Occam's razor — credited to a 14th-century English philosopher — which suggests that the simplest explanation is usually the correct one. In medicine, it favors a single unifying diagnosis over multiple separate ones. While this tenet of parsimony may not hold in adults with multiple comorbidities, it generally applies to otherwise healthy children. So far, Jane was the exception.

I dig deeper into her history and uncover some enlightening new details. Jane is a sporty fifth grader who started soccer at six but had to quit after a hip injury. She loves gymnastics — and she's really bendy. How does that all connect? A hyperflexible (i.e., hypermobile) kid with a clotting deficiency, recurrent post-tonsillectomy bleeds, and frequent nosebleeds? Suddenly, the pieces start to shift into place.

EDS. That's it!

Ehlers-Danlos Syndrome (EDS) is a genetic disorder affecting the connective tissues and weakening the walls of blood vessels. It has many forms but can cause joint hypermobility and instability, in addition to fragility of blood vessels. When EDS and VWD occur together, it's the perfect storm. Throw in an inciting event like tonsillectomy surgery and voilà! It's a bloodbath.

After a bit of work, Jane's nosebleed is controlled with gentle packing and a squirtable hemostatic foam called Floseal. She's calm and her labs are ok. If I leave now, I think I can make it back for the end of the fourth period …

I burst in through the gym's side door just as she shoots, just as she scores.

She thinks I'm still gone but I see her scanning the crowd anyway.

When she pivots back around, she catches my eye.

Then, she smiles, full-metal braces showing.

Later, on the ride home, Scarlett is a combination of elated and mildly annoyed.

"You promised you'd stay for the whole thing … Of course, I understand though."

"I know. I know I did. Something really important came up. I'm so sorry … but I came back."

"But did you see it Mommy? Did you really see my shot?"

I search her eyes — desperately — for that look. That wounded look of Dr. Burgess's daughter.

And, to my great relief, it's not there.

"Yes, Scarlett. I'm so proud of you. I absolutely did."

CHAPTER 12

THE EXIT PROCEDURE

SOME SURGERIES ARE so mind-blowing they sound like
science fiction. The Ex-Utero Intrapartum Treatment (EXIT)
procedure is one of them. It's typically the only viable option
when a baby has a known or suspected airway obstruction that
would prevent breathing immediately after birth — often due to
a congenital anomaly compressing or blocking the upper airway.
Without this method, the baby would suffocate once separated
from the placental oxygen supply. In this carefully choreographed
operation, the baby is partially delivered but remains connected to
the placenta via the umbilical cord, allowing continued oxygenation
through the mother's circulation while the surgical team works to
secure the airway. It's not a guaranteed fix — complications can
threaten both mother and baby — but sometimes, it's their only
chance at survival.

Planning an EXIT procedure requires seamless collaboration
across multiple specialties. Obstetric anesthesia, pediatric anesthesia, maternal-fetal medicine (MFM), obstetrics, neonatology,
pediatric surgery, and pediatric otolaryngology each play defined
roles, with one person from every team designated as "in charge."

These complex surgeries are typically performed only at major medical centers. In the lead-up to D-day (delivery day), teams hold planning meetings, run simulations, and work through exhaustive checklists. The goal is to anticipate problems before they happen — because when the wheels fall off, you need a plan to keep from careening into the concrete divider.

Planning an EXIT procedure requires seamless collaboration across multiple specialties.

Dr. Eve McCrory is our Residency Director. Originally from Connecticut, she joined our hospital two years ago after a decade of practicing in Tennessee. It's always a strange transition when a near-contemporary becomes your division "boss." Lucky for me, Eve has navigated the shift with grace and respect for us OGs — the original gangsters of the ENT department. She's smart, strong-willed, and practical like me, though a bit more cautious. As she likes to remind me, "Tali, I saw a lot of bad shit down there."

We recently bonded over our shared love of *Shetland*, a BBC crime show set unsurprisingly in the Shetland Isles, known for its dramatic landscapes, rich wildlife, and Viking history. While I became so enamored with the show — and its stunning scenery — that Alex and I traveled there last summer on a full-blown fan holiday, I think Eve just thought it was a "really cool setting."

Eve has been working closely with the MFM team and has laid out a meticulous plan. In this case, a bulky neck mass was identified on prenatal ultrasound and further characterized by fetal MRI. Its appearance suggested a teratoma — a tumor that arises from stem cells and can contain almost any type of body tissue: skin, hair, teeth, you name it. A cervical (neck) teratoma is a very rare congenital tumor. These masses can grow quite large in utero and are often disfiguring. In some extreme cases, they become so enormous it looks as if the baby has a second head. The primary concern is that the mass will compress the airway so severely after birth that the baby won't be able to take its first breath. To prevent this, a plan is made to secure the airway immediately at delivery — through a scheduled, surgical birth. The mass is excised at a later time.

In this case, the MFM team schedules an induction at 38 weeks' gestation, giving us four weeks to prepare. Still, I suspect that this baby is going to crash the party before its assigned birthday. The mother has already been admitted more than once for pregnancy-related issues. It's a delicate balance — trying to get the fetus to term while avoiding a middle-of-the-night emergency.

I suspect that this baby is going to crash the party before its assigned birthday.

Unfortunately, my sixth sense is right. On Monday, just as I start my long clinic day, I get the call from Eve.

"You need to come. She's in labor."

"Like now, or do I have some time?"

"Now."

I peek around the corner at my packed waiting room and know I'm about to piss off an already-angry crowd. But I have no choice.

I grab my bag and walk out into the sea of eager parents and their children. Everyone looks up.

"I'm so sorry but there is an emergency with an unborn child at The Medical Center. I *have* to go."

I rush out the door without turning my head to witness the fury in my wake.

I know that speeding to the hospital and getting into an accident on the way won't help anyone, so I have a strict rule against it. Still, from the moment I arrive, I'm sprinting through the parking lot and changing into my scrubs like Superwoman without the phone booth. Mildly out of shape, I reach the OR desk huffing and puffing — not exactly the classic picture of a superhero. Naturally, it's a ghost town.

This was a deeply desired pregnancy. After three rounds of in vitro fertilization (IVF), the parents were overjoyed to finally conceive. They celebrated passing the 15-week mark — only to be blindsided by the discovery of a "mass." The rest of the pregnancy was clouded by fear and uncertainty. What would their child look like? How would it breathe? Would it survive?

The pregnancy was clouded by fear and uncertainty. What would their child look like? How would it breathe? Would it survive?

A key ethical dilemma in the EXIT procedure is the risk to the mother — most notably, the potential for life-threatening blood loss. Another serious possibility is the need for an emergency hysterectomy. In the worst-case scenario, the baby may not survive, and the mother may lose her ability to carry another child. Like so much in medicine, the risks and benefits must be weighed with care. It's an enormous decision for the parents, and no amount of counseling can truly ease that burden.

After an initial lull, suddenly the OR hallway feels like game day at the Super Bowl — the whole place is buzzing. Two of the pediatric anesthesiologists, Dr. Kathy Gruffy and Dr. Isabel Pesola, have made sticky name tags for everyone to attach to their surgical caps for easy identification. I slap mine on. It reads: "Peds ENT."

Inside the cavernous operating room, each specialty has claimed its own space. Eve and I are tucked into the far-right pocket. One by one, the teams complete their individual "pre-flight checks." We've got multiple instrument trays laid out — ranging from the "This isn't so bad ..." setup to the one labeled "Damn! We need an open tracheotomy."

Once everyone is ready, the mother is brought into the operating room. To avoid bedlam, the teams enter in coordinated shifts. First up is obstetric anesthesia — they place the epidural and then induce general anesthesia. By the time we're called in, the mother is already intubated. The scrub nurse is preparing the sterile table where the baby will be placed.

This shit is getting REAL.

Time-Out

This is a 34-week-gestation fetus with a large neck mass thought to be a teratoma that is obstructing the airway. The plan is for an EXIT procedure. The baby will be partially delivered and then placed on a table between the mother's legs with the umbilical cord attached. Anesthesia will continue to medicate and resuscitate the mother while we (the pediatric ENT team) will attempt to expose the larynx and intubate the child. If this is not successful, we will proceed to tracheostomy to establish a surgical airway. The neck mass will be resected later, in conjunction with pediatric surgery.

The uterus is wide open, and the obstetricians are working to deliver the baby safely while minimizing blood loss for the mother. Ideally, dependence on maternal-fetal circulation should be limited to 30 minutes or less. Beyond that, the risk of uterine atony increases. Uterine atony occurs when the uterus fails to contract effectively after childbirth, leaving the extensive uterine blood vessel system open. It can happen naturally after prolonged labor or, as in this case, because of intentionally maintaining blood flow to the baby after delivery. If not treated promptly, it can lead to life-threatening hemorrhage.

Eve and I are standing on opposite sides of the OR table with bated breath. We're both hot under our scrubs despite the frigidity of the room.

"Start the clock."

As soon as the baby is delivered, he is handed to us. I ignore the wildly twisted features and attempt to intubate the baby's airway using the standard technique. It doesn't work. Eve attempts a second technique. It, too, doesn't work.

"Twenty-five minutes."

The mass is too obstructive. We need to open the neck. We need to do it NOW.

Eve and I don't have much operating history between us, but it doesn't matter. Like me, she's seasoned. We'll quickly find our rhythm.

It's go-time.

Surgery Start Time — 2:55 p.m.

We work in unison, quickly and efficiently. Our senior resident lifts the mass off to the side so we can identify any recognizable landmarks. Normal anatomy is shifted out of place from the tumor. Still, we stick to the basics.

Feel the sternal notch.

Slide down to the cricoid ring.

Palpate the thyroid notch.

Two fingerbreadths above … and … begin.

The 15-blade slices through the skin, then dermis, then soft subcutaneous tissue.

"Twenty minutes."

Gotta find the midline.

The clock is ticking.

Mom is losing blood.

These two vulnerable lives in our hands, balanced on a knife's edge.

"Eighteen minutes."

We find the right spot, cut through the cartilaginous rings, and the telltale mucous bubbles out.

We suction and see the beautiful hollow of the airway.

"3.0 trach, please."

"Fifteen minutes."

Eve inserts the plastic tube into the space. It looks wildly off-kilter, but we know it's right.

The glorious yellow waves of carbon dioxide appear on the monitor, followed by the peaked blue waves of oxygen saturation, reassuring us of proper gas exchange.

"We are in! Clamp the cord."

The OB team returns to working on the mom. The cord is clamped, and they begin closing the uterus.

The timer is stopped.

This is just the beginning ...

Once the infant is stabilized, we go out to the waiting room, searching for the father. The mother is still under general anesthesia. She hasn't met her baby yet.

Dad is shifting back and forth, wringing his hands. He looks lost.

"Congratulations on your new baby. Your son is doing well. Due to the large size of the mass, we did have to secure an airway through his neck."

Dad's pupils dilate, his brow furrows, but he doesn't respond.

"Your wife is doing well. The doctors are still working on her, but she is not bleeding, and she did not require a hysterectomy."

He remains stoic.

"Do you want to see him?"

He nods but does not move initially. We lead him gently toward the NICU.

We stop in front of the isolette labeled "Baby Smith." Inside is a fresh new baby boy with a button nose, adorable ears, and light eyes. The left side of his face is perfect — with rounded cheeks and full lips, but the right side is Picasso-esque. The skin is stretched taut and thinly draped over the tumor with spider blue veins branching outward in a starburst pattern.

Dad's eyes widen, tears threatening to spill down his face.

"Will … he … always …look like that?"

They name him Jackson, after his grandfather, a former lieutenant colonel in the Army who received two purple hearts for bravery in WWII.

Days later, we reconvene in OR 1. It's time for step two: resection of the teratoma.

TIME-OUT

This is a 2-day-old male delivered via EXIT procedure with a surgical airway established at birth who is here for resection of a large cervical teratoma. Drs. Lando and McCrory from Peds ENT and Dr. Dylan Stewart, chief of Peds Surgery, are collaborating. Dr. Mike Yao will scrub in as needed for nerve dissection. There are two units of blood on hold to the OR and two more units in the blood bank. The patient will have nerve monitoring throughout.

A teratoma is like a giant tissue expander, stretching, distorting, and displacing all the normal structures around it. As a result, nothing is where it should be. This makes it hard to remove without damaging something important, like the many nerves and vessels in the vicinity. Another challenge is deciding where to make the incision and how much skin to remove. You must picture in your mind's eye what will be … in the future … when everything heals and settles. This kind of surgery requires imagination in addition to skill.

With the baby lying supine on the operating table, we draw a line that we envision to be a future skin crease, to create a favorable scar. This long incision is delineated with a purple marker. The newborn is hooked up to a special intraoperative nerve-monitoring system. We prepare the patient with careful attention to sterility. We cut through the layers of paper-thin skin and muscle. We try to minimize the risks, but the tumor can be so intertwined with other structures that injury is not always avoidable.

The three of us take turns dissecting the mass from its surrounding attachments. A portion of it ducks deep under the muscles of the neck, toward the trachea. There's bleeding, which is expected in a tumor with such an abundant blood supply, but we get hemostatic control. Mike steps in to lend his special head-and-neck expertise. He dissects the tumor carefully off the recurrent laryngeal nerve, which controls the movement of the vocal cord. The monitor jumps to life, beeping repeatedly. This means we're in the danger zone for injury. With careful technique, he preserves the nerve. Although there is always a risk of "stretch injury" (a temporary weakness of the nerve, which may eventually return to normal function), it appears unharmed. We continue dissecting, surrounding and freeing the tumor from its attachments. The marginal mandibular nerve is a fine branch of the facial nerve in these infants. It controls the muscle to the lower lip. It is very susceptible to injury. We aim to avoid it, but it's so wispy that it's nearly impossible to identify.

After a few collaborative hours, we are finally ready to "deliver the tumor." We hand it over to Hannah, our capable scrub nurse (and one of the cherished few who will always stay and do overtime for me with heart). It weighs nearly three pounds. She cutely nicknames it "Tim the teratoma."

Once the wound is fastidiously closed, Dylan, Mike, Eve and I leave the OR. We find Jackson's parents encircled by an entire Irish clan of relatives.

"The surgery went well. Jackson lost some blood and, not unexpectedly, needed a transfusion. But he's stable and in recovery."

Before we know it, we're being clobbered with hugs from various appreciative family members. As usual, Mike has craftily ducked out of the tumult — he's definitely not a hugger. Eve and I, on the other hand, are a bit slower with the reflexes. We get nailed with a series of unsolicited squeezes and smooches.

"He'll be swollen, but it will calm down over the next several weeks. His cry may be weak initially and he may have some trouble swallowing, which we will monitor, but we believe the laryngeal nerve was preserved. The marginal nerve is always unpredictable. He may very well have a slight asymmetry to his smile. Time will tell."

"But he's ok. You said he's ok."

"Yes. He is."

LATER

When Jackson comes in for his one-year follow-up, he's already toddling around and looking for trouble.

"Hieeee!" he smiles widely.

In seconds, he takes off running with impunity. His tracheostomy tube was successfully removed a few weeks after his surgery. His raspiness and initial noisy breathing resulting from a stretched laryngeal nerve — as well as structural weakness of the trachea (called tracheomalacia) — has resolved. His incision is well-healed and nicely hidden.

Handsome and chubby with a sweep of sandy brown hair, his voice is loud and clear. He's destined to be a charmer, for sure. He has two perfect dimples and cat-green eyes with yellow rims. But the most adorable thing about him is that perfectly imperfect smile.

DEBRIEF

"In these cases, preservation of the mother's life always comes before the fetus."

"When it comes to the pediatric patients, we are a team. Egos are left at the door."

"If you can't get it done, maybe someone else can. Swallow your pride. Call for help; hell ... call in the cavalry if they'll come. Alternatively, as in this case, defer to your second in command if you have one. That's the benefit of back-up."

"If there is potential for chaos, anticipatory organization is key."

"When many teams are involved, a defined hierarchy is necessary for clarity. Who is in charge? What are the goals? Which of them takes ultimate priority? What are the expectations and benchmarks for success?"

"Be eager to learn from others. Listen closely for any tips or tricks."

"At the end of the day, the only important thing is that the patients receive the best care."

AT HOME

It's amazing how efficient I can be at the hospital, while otherwise I get totally bogged down. What should I do first anyway? Clean the garage or organize the mudroom? Is it worth organizing the pantry when the kids will mess it up again anyway? When one daughter outgrows her clothing, should I move the bin to the younger daughter's closet or store it in the attic? What if the girls are two sizes apart?

Sometimes, I get so overwhelmed with the preciousness of my free time that I am paralyzed with indecision. Should I surprise Scarlett with an unexpected pick-up from school, or should I be in the basement sorting out the school supplies? Is it best to treat myself to a spontaneous pedicure or should I update the expired car inspection? Maybe I should just take a quick nap …

Similarly, I can rearrange my operative schedule like a jigsaw puzzle, but I'm total shit at arranging multiple carpools. This isn't just a matter of focus. I actually cannot do it. My friend Karen is the complete opposite. She's a super-impressive lawyer with a million balls in the air just like me but she's like a circus juggler with the household stuff too. I've seen her make a grid that enables her to drive her son Isaac to hockey, daughter Jordana to and from a doctor's appointment, and her other daughter Nava to a bat mitzvah in different towns at the same time on the same day. Meanwhile, I end up forgetting to pick up Scarlett from her basketball clinic, leave Juliette with no ride home from afterschool, and miss Milla's endocrine appointment that I already rescheduled three months ago (but forgot to put on the family calendar app … again).

I am aware that, from the outside, some people mistakenly assume that I have it together. I don't. There are constant fumbles — lots of tears, and endless apologies to my kids, my husband, my hairdresser, and my dentist (especially). I've leaned heavily on friends, hired help, nannies, au pairs … you name it. Women — like Rhonda (my saint), Malka (my rock), Ilana (my psychologist), Lauren and Deena (my doctors), and Avigail (my problem solver) — have come through with unreciprocated carpool rides, last-minute birthday decorations I never return, and emergency vanilla coffee creamer at 8:00 a.m. on a Saturday. I'm at least three years behind on bar and bat mitzvah gifts. Some of these kids will probably be married before I catch up. On more than one occasion, when I've been stuck in the OR, my neighbors Grace and Louis have picked up my daughter from the bus stop — usually after I suddenly realize she's alone, locked out of the house, has no cell phone, and it's raining. Traditionally, I've relied on Karen to remind me when to sign up for every sport or prep course (driver's ed, ACT, etc.) imaginable, and Debbie for all things school-schedule-related — until her kids switched schools, and then I was screwed. Over the years, I've leaned upon so many people for so many things.

The best reciprocity I can offer is otolaryngologic medical advice, the occasional night-and-weekend prescription service, and the deepest, most exhausted gratitude my tired soul can muster. Oh — and countless unsolicited, detailed, and (to me, at least) utterly fascinating stories — like Jackson's — to distract them from my never-ending fuck-ups.

Over the years, I've leaned upon so many people for so many things. The best reciprocity I can offer is otolaryngologic medical advice, the occasional night-and-weekend prescription service, and the deepest, most exhausted gratitude my tired soul can muster.

CHAPTER 13

WHEN THE WALLS
CAVE IN

WHILE SUCCESSES IN medicine are easy to celebrate, it's the failures — and the patients who don't prevail — that can bring you to your knees. These are the cases that take hold of you, preoccupy your thoughts, fill you with self-doubt, and shake you to your bones. Henry J. was that patient for me.

When I first met Henry John James Murphy, III, he was a tiny thing with a big name. Born at just 26 weeks, he was a twin who weighed 1 pound 9 ounces — intubated, ventilated, and extremely fragile. In those early days, his parents' only hope was survival. His mom spent her days sitting between the two isolettes, riding the relentless waves of pulmonary hypertension and bronchopulmonary dysplasia — two common but daunting complications in premature infants. While Henry's twin, Anabella Joy Grace, began to thrive, most of the updates about Henry were consistently grim.

Your baby has a 50% chance of survival.
Your baby has a brain bleed.
Your baby's lungs are not expanding.

Your baby has a 50% chance of a normal life.

From there, it didn't get better.

Your baby's immature gut is failing … we need to do surgery.
Your baby's heart has a hole … we need to do surgery.
Your baby's underdeveloped lungs are not maturing … we need to do surgery.

This is where I came into Henry's life. The plastic container that held him was covered in blue adornments with a bedazzled name plate and augmented with countless family photos. Inside his temperature-controlled, sound-reducing, infection-protecting home, he sported an adorable hand-crocheted light blue hat. His mom, Tracy, sobbed uncontrollably as I detailed my need to transition him from the taped oral tube to one surgically inserted into his teeny neck.

After his tracheostomy and g-tube placement, Henry remained too medically precarious to be cared for at home. He was moved to the children's rehabilitation facility near the hospital, where he remained for many months. I began to see him regularly in my outpatient clinic. I watched him grow, then slowly graduate from a state of constant instability. Over the course of the following years, the once unfathomable occurred. Henry was weaned off the ventilator, then off pressurized oxygen and, ultimately, began to breathe completely on his own.

At this point, all ex-NICU parents seem to share one unifying goal: to get the trach out. This milestone — known as decannulation — is the process of removing a child's tracheostomy tube. While the act itself is deceptively simple (you just take the tube out), the real challenge is making sure it's safe to do so. The first step in assessing readiness for decannulation is an airway evaluation in the operating room.

TIME-OUT

This is a 2.5-year-old ex-26-week-preemie who has a long-term tracheostomy and is here for a direct laryngoscopy and bronchoscopy to determine his eligibility for a decannulation trial.

For most airway surgeons, the setup for an airway evaluation is regimented and methodical. Even the orientation of the operating table (precisely 90 degrees), the placement of the specific metal wheeling table with ledges (to the surgeon's right), and the light source (just behind and slightly to the left of me) are all predetermined. Unlike the mayhem of emergency cases, these are moments where I insist on exact preparation. I repeat the required checklist and its precise layout until it becomes a routine irreversibly etched into the minds of all my trainees — or at least, it should be.

A survey of the airway for this purpose proceeds systematically from top to bottom. First, we examine the supraglottis — the upper part of the larynx above the vocal cords. Next, we assess the vocal cords themselves, focusing on their appearance and mobility. Deeper still, we evaluate the caliber of the subglottis, the narrowest part of a child's airway and the most prone to swelling or scarring. Finally, we assess the trachea — all the way down to the carina, the point where the trachea (windpipe) divides into the two main bronchi, each leading to a lung — for structural integrity and signs of floppiness. Each of these elements plays a critical role in determining whether Henry can breathe normally.

Tracy brings Henry into the room and attaches the tubing with anesthetic gas flowing. She is gentle and soothing, with genuine warmth.

"Ok, mama, give him a kiss on the cheek," Tracy is then escorted out to the waiting room.

SURGERY START TIME — THURSDAY, 8:30 A.M.

With Henry's neck in extension, a blue half-sheet is laid across his body.

"Towel for the head. 2-inch plastic tape to secure, no towel clip. Tooth guard. Ball-tip suction attached, power on medium high."

"Down the right gutter, swipe the tongue all the way to the left. Tell me when you're in the vallecula and you can see the laryngeal inlet."

"I'm there, Dr. Lando."

"Spray the cords with lidocaine. Suction the mucous. Defog your scope. Show me your best view."

The thumb-shaped flap of the cartilaginous epiglottis sticks up vertically. The vocal cords open and close rhythmically with each breath.

"Cord motion looks good. Go on through."

My wonderful resident, Maria, deftly advances the telescope to reveal the surprisingly pristine circular anatomy of the subglottis. Maria is sharp, funny, and a personal fav of mine (shh ... don't tell anyone).

"No stenosis. Given his prolonged intubation, this is great news. Now, let's look at the peristomal area."

"I will pull out the trach. Isabel, we're going to disconnect the circuit for a minute."

She nods her permission, and we proceed.

Although this segment of airway doesn't look perfect, it doesn't look too compromised either. We complete the assessment of the remainder of the lower trachea and first branches of the bronchial tree. All appears normal.

"Not bad. This airway may work for him."

I use a knife and scissors to freshen the edges of the stoma hole to promote healing and replace the trach with a smaller diameter tube.

Afterward, I find Tracy and tell her the good news.

"We're going to admit Henry for a capping trial. Fingers crossed."

She is so happy, she cries. This is the news she's been hoping for. Henry is admitted with a plan to test his ability to breathe overnight with the tracheostomy covered. If he passes this initial "capping trial," the tracheostomy tube will be removed in the morning. If all goes well, he'll remain in the hospital for at least one more day of observation to monitor for any issues.

Over the next 48 hours, Henry does great. The tracheostomy tube is removed, and an occlusive dressing is placed to cover the stoma (hole). On the day of discharge, I find him in the playroom — sporting a perfectly gelled mini-mohawk and a striped blue-green shirt. He is breathing comfortably, and cheerfully coloring with crayons. Tracy is ecstatic.

"I can't wait to take him swimming with his sister."

"We'll get there."

Henry is sent home with a plan to follow up with me in two weeks.

It's Wednesday evening as I strap Junie and Evie into their matching neon-yellow reflector harnesses for a walk. It's one of those rare weekday nights when it's still light out, even after my workday ends. A gentle, warm breeze brushes past — the kind I crave during cold Northeastern winters. Just as I step outside, a text chimes from my answering service. It doesn't sound good.

> *Emergency Call*
>
> *Patient: Henry John James Murphy*
>
> *Caller: Tracy Murphy*
>
> *Message: Henry isn't breathing normally. He's making a strange whistling noise, and his neck is sucking in. Please call.*

I dial the number, but I already know what's wrong. Henry's stoma has closed, and he isn't tolerating it. He needs to come back to the emergency room immediately. I am going to have to tell Tracy exactly what she doesn't want to hear. I turn the dogs back around and head back toward the garage ...

When Henry arrives to the ED less than an hour later, he is working really hard to breathe. His smile is gone. His hair is disheveled. Tracy is worried. Her smile has faded too.

I don't sugarcoat it.

"I need to put the tracheostomy back in."

I expect a barrage of tears, pleading, and negotiation. But Tracy surprises me.

"I know."

Surgery Start Time —
Wednesday, 10:00 p.m.

A 4.0 ventilating bronchoscope is introduced into Henry's airway. Soon, the camera reveals a 1-centimeter segment where the tracheal walls appear buckled — like the frame of a house caving in. The critical narrowing at the stoma site (the opening into the trachea) forms an acute angle. The anterior tracheal rings have lost their structural integrity and collapsed inward. It must have happened as soon as the overlying skin sealed shut.

"It's a pretty significant A-frame deformity. There's no choice. We need to re-open the hole. He's going to need an airway reconstruction surgery."

I inject the closed stoma site with lidocaine and epinephrine (my typical cocktail for these cases) to numb the area and reduce bleeding. Then, the standard steps.

"15-blade. Tracheal dilator. Suction. 4.0 pediatric uncuffed tracheostomy."

"It's in. Ok, folks, let's wrap it up."

Once again, Tracy takes the news better than I expect. We talk through what a laryngotracheal reconstruction will mean for Henry — the multiple steps involved, the potential timing (which she wants to be immediate), the risks, and the chances of success. To honor her wish, I make the difficult decision to cancel more than 30 patients scheduled for the following day.

TIME-OUT

This is a 2.5-year-old male, recently decannulated, who returned to the ED yesterday in extremis after his stoma closed. We are here today to perform a laryngotracheal reconstruction using either a rib or thyroid cartilage graft. We will prep the right chest and neck separately.

Once asleep, Henry is intubated from above and the tracheostomy removed. A marking pen is used to mark the future inframammary (below the breast) crease on his right side, approximately two centimeters in length. The area is prepped and draped in the usual sterile fashion. The neck incision is marked and prepped in a similar fashion.

After the muscles are divided and the anterior airway is completely skeletonized, there is an obvious gap that must be bridged with donor cartilage. This can be taken from the ear, neck, or rib. This additional support is necessary to provide enough structural integrity to keep the airway open.

RECONSTRUCTIVE SURGERY START TIME — FRIDAY, 9:00 A.M.

"Calipers."

I carefully measure the dimensions of the defect.

"11 x 6 millimeters. Please write it down."

This is the minimum length of donor cartilage necessary. Weighing the pros and cons, we decide to harvest rib because of its superior strength.

"10-blade. Double-prong skin hooks. Tonsil clamp. Bovie."

I dissect through skin and muscle, exposing the sixth rib. Carefully avoiding vessels and nerves, I cut across the superior border of the rib, through the thin, pale-pink layer of perichondrium. This part of the surgery is delicate. The goal is to harvest a healthy piece of cartilage with the superficial lining attached, while leaving the inner perichondrial layer intact. Slip even slightly too deep, and you risk puncture — causing a pneumothorax, or collapsed lung. That's a problem we definitely don't need today.

"Doyen."

The doyen retractor is a funny-looking instrument with a slightly spiraled hook shape that looks like a curly metal French fry. I feel a sense of relief as it glides easily under the rib, enabling me to cut down on its flat surface with impunity.

"Wrap this in Telfa gauze and guard it with your life."

I hand the prized specimen to Christian, and he transfers it gently to the back table in preparation for carving.

Next, we will fashion the graft with a knife on a white stone carving block, place it in the neck, and secure it in place with sutures.

The remainder of the case proceeds smoothly. Once the graft is sutured in place, we test the site for an air leak and there is none.

We close the wound in multiple layers, stitch in drains, and cover the neck and chest with sterile dressings.

Henry is transferred to the ICU in stable condition. I find his parents and accompany them up the elevator to the PICU waiting room.

"Everything went wonderfully. Hopefully we will return to the OR in four days to remove the tube and confirm that the graft is healing well."

On POD (post-op day) 1 and 2, the wound looks great.

Then, what began as resounding success soon begins to fail.

What began as resounding success soon begins to fail.

On POD 3, on morning rounds, my resident reports scant murky drainage from the neck site. The surrounding skin still appears healthy and there are no foreboding signs of trapped air. Fingers crossed ... everything is still ok.

By POD 4, the skin becomes discolored and patchy. Henry spikes a fever. The drain output increases and darkens. A sample is sent to the lab. When I palpate his neck, I detect the alarming crackles of crepitus.

"The wound is infected." This is *not* ok.

"What does that mean?" Tracy asks.

"It's not a good sign. We'll try conservative management. Start daily peroxide irrigations and broaden his antibiotic coverage. We'll see what the cultures reveal."

Tracy goes silent, burying her head in her hands.

Several days later, my text pings.

Dr. Lando. It's fungus.

My heart sinks. Fungus — the death knell of autologous grafts. It's often worse than nasty bacteria, signaling not only infection but also the breakdown of healthy tissue.

From there, the downward spiral continues.

We need to go back in.

After days of sleeplessness and isolation, Tracy becomes hysterical — wailing and inconsolable.

"Why? Why me? You promised. I won't go back to before. I just can't. I won't."

"I need to do this. Henry needs me to do this. I don't know what I will find, but whatever it is, we need to deal with it."

I have to call for help to pry Tracy's grip from my arm. She will not stop yelling.

We enlist the help of the psychiatric team to settle her down. It takes another hour of persuasion before she finally relents. Then, she signs the consent for: *Airway evaluation and wound wash-out. Possible replacement of tracheostomy.*

SURGERY START TIME — SUNDAY, 10:00 A.M.

The wound looks terrible from the start. It opens way too easily, pulling apart with just a gentle tug. Inside, there's softness and inflammation where there should be strength and epithelialization — the critical phase of wound healing in which new epithelial cells (skin or mucosal lining) grow and spread to cover the surface. We thoroughly debride the wound, surgically removing dead or damaged tissue, then irrigate it with an antibiotic-laden solution. We poke and prod the reconstructed surface. To my elation, underneath the debris, most of the graft is intact. On first inspection of the airway surface, I can almost believe there is nothing wrong.

But I know better. When it comes to these things, where there is smoke, there is fire. The tension in my neck does not release. Somewhere in here is failure. After multiple delicate manipulations, I lift up a small piece of tissue and telltale bubbles trickle to the surface.

On first inspection of the airway surface, I can almost believe there is nothing wrong. But I know better.

"There it is. It's just this corner bit that's leaking air. But it's enough."

I cut a tiny wedge of unhealthy cartilage.

Will it hold? Or will it all fall apart, leaving a gaping hole?

Should I remove the entire graft, give up for now, and replace the trach?

Should I start over and harvest another rib?

Or should I take a chance … wait and see how it heals?

The multitude of options swirl in my head.

This is where decades of experience count, where the science of medicine becomes an art. This is where I thank G-d for camaraderie. This is where I phone a friend.

"Can you talk?"

"Whatcha got?"

I quickly run through the details, the evolution of the problem, and the current state of affairs.

"If it's just a small corner, it can hold. The body should granulate the hole. One can never be sure, but it's worth a shot."

From your lips to G-d's ears. Cross my fingers. Throw salt over my left shoulder.

Back in the PICU, Henry remains sedated and intubated. Further days pass by.

Every day, the wound is checked and rechecked. Each morning, I hold my breath for good news ... or bad.

Then, finally, one fine day, the sun begins to shine. Henry's fevers subside, his lab tests normalize, and his skin takes on a healthy hue. The drain output drops to a minimum. One afternoon — after what feels like forever, but has been exactly 10 days — I say, "It's time. He's as ready as he'll ever be."

I stand at the bedside biting my nails as the nurse prepares to remove the intubation tube. I am fixated on Henry's neck, his chest, and the tone and values on the monitors.

Please. Let it be good.

The tube is removed.

And ... then ... Henry breathes.

LATER (AND AN EXPLANATION)

Keeping a child sedated with a tube in place during prolonged critical illness requires extended use of sedatives and narcotics. When these medications are stopped abruptly or weaned too quickly, post-extubation withdrawal can occur. The challenge is that each patient responds differently to medication titration — there's no universal formula. Ex-preemies are particularly difficult to manage, as many have developed a tolerance during infancy.

This necessitates higher doses of benzodiazepines and opioids to keep them still. The weaning process can be lengthy, often involving several weeks of methadone tapers. Even with careful planning, withdrawal can still occur. Respiratory distress is a common symptom, which adds to the diagnostic challenge in children with underlying airway issues.

Henry was brutal to sedate, requiring IV doses that could tranquilize a bull elephant. The volume of fluid needed to run these medications led to fluid overload. His face grew puffy, and his hands and feet swelled. This triggered the use of diuretics to clear the excess fluid, which then dried him out so much that he needed additional medications just to maintain his blood pressure.

It was not so surprising that Tracy developed ICU-family delirium. The extreme stress and emotional strain of watching her child in critical condition caused mood swings and severe anxiety. The constant alarms and uncertainty, coupled with sleep deprivation, left her irritable and often irrational. Levelheaded conversation and decision making with the care team became nearly impossible.

Even with the support of family, friends, and her professional psychologist who consulted over the phone, Tracy's demands became as difficult to manage as Henry's medical condition. This led to further staff frustration and fatigue.

Tracy's demands became as difficult to manage as Henry's medical condition

Ultimately, ever so gradually across several weeks, the tide did turn. Just as impossibly as he had descended into darkness, sweet Henry began to re-emerge.

And then, on a mid-summer morning, he was ready to leave the hospital … without a hole in his neck … healed.

DEBRIEF

"Never make promises you can't keep. Don't even imply them."

"Nevertheless, you will find that even if you don't, your patients or their parents may believe you did."

"Understand, people are afraid and looking to you for assurance."

"Just because they want that surety, doesn't mean you can give it, no matter how badly you wish you could."

"When it's necessary, be assertive and confident, but never cocky."

"Your life as a surgeon will be a mixture of so many elements you can and cannot control. Accept that."

"When things go wrong, be clear. Do not hide from the truth. It will find you anyway."

"Even if the news is bad, break it down for the family. Look them directly in the eyes and give it to them straight."

"Setbacks occur. They are an occupational hazard. Still, never try to bury failure."

"When what you do properly fails, do not give up. Just take a bit of time. Learn from it. Quickly lick your wounds. Then, buck up, regroup, and try again."

AT HOME

Although I had begun to lose hope that Henry would ever heal, in the end, his body found a way. The process was protracted and took its toll on him, on his mother, and even on me. It highlighted the inextricable duality of pediatric medicine, in which there is not only the patient and their ailment, but also a vulnerable parent (or parents) too. Though the mechanics of surgery are formally taught, the psychology of being a doctor is not. It is gleaned by instinct, exposure, situation, and reflection.

Though the mechanics of surgery are formally taught, the psychology of being a doctor is not. It is gleaned by instinct, exposure, situation, and reflection.

Henry's happy ending was complicated and full of consequence. Despite the ultimate victory — breathing on his own — uncertainty still lingered. Delayed from his ex-preemie days, Henry had only recently begun to speak, eat by mouth, and run around like a typical toddler before his surgeries. Weeks of sedation and immobility erased those hard-earned milestones. It took months of occupational, feeding, and speech therapy to regain what was lost. Slowly, Henry began moving forward — back toward the place where he had once started.

For my part, I walked away from the experience battered and bruised — but wiser. Despite the emotional toll and drawn-out course, I was fortunate to have faithful colleagues in the thick of it with me — encouraging me, steadying me. They remind me that Henry's setbacks and his mother's emotional struggles were a force majeure, not something I could have predicted or controlled. Beyond those in my immediate sphere, I was — and still am — immeasurably blessed to have people who always answer my calls, listen (repeatedly), and offer guidance, no matter how swamped they are themselves.

And, most of all, I was fortunate enough to see Henry all the way through, to the other side.

AS THE WORLD
SHUT DOWN

IN THE LATE winter of 2020, the SARS-CoV-2 virus — and its resulting respiratory illness, COVID-19 — began to unleash devastation across the globe. As the disease spread at alarming rates, it was a frightening time to be a physician. It was especially terrifying to be a surgeon who specializes in the airway. As otolaryngologists, we were exposed to particularly high viral loads from a disease transmitted via aerosolized particles. At first, we were even instructed not to wear masks, out of concern that it might "scare our patients." For a time, we continued treating patients as usual in our offices, which required close-contact examinations. In those early days, so much was still unknown or misunderstood. Hospital policies often lagged behind the rapidly evolving reality.

During this highly uncertain time, Chloe was born at a small community hospital in the Catskill Mountains. Immediately after delivery, she was noted to have abnormal-sounding breathing and intermittent "blue spells." About two weeks before all our hospital units closed to outside transfers, Chloe was transported to our NICU by ambulance. I happened to be in the hospital that day — operating.

In between a frenuloplasty (a tongue-tie release) and the excision of a branchial cleft fistula (a surgery for a congenital neck abnormality), my team and I gathered at Chloe's bedside for a consultation.

When Chloe was asleep, she appeared relatively peaceful — her breathing more of a hum than a distress call. The trouble came when she was awake and upset; she simply couldn't manage. The hollow of her neck would deepen with suprasternal retractions, her nostrils would flare, and her tiny body would heave. Her oxygen levels would plummet, and her lips would turn a dusky purple. Then, just as quickly, she'd recover. A flexible scope exam revealed that her vocal cords could not abduct (open) more than 1 millimeter, though they retained normal ability to adduct (close).

Congenital (or neonatal) vocal fold paralysis — when the vocal cords do not move properly — is the second most common cause of noisy breathing in newborns. In most cases, the etiology is idiopathic, meaning the cause is unknown. The immobile vocal fold may be on one side or both. When paralysis is bilateral, the infant becomes functionally restricted. While they may appear stable when calm, they cannot meet basic physical demands like crying or feeding.

Sometimes, vocal fold paralysis is part of a broader genetic syndrome. Other times, as in Chloe's case, it presents as an isolated finding in an otherwise healthy newborn. An MRI is typically ordered to rule out neurologic causes that may be treatable — such as a Chiari malformation, in which compression of the brainstem affects the vagus nerves responsible for vocal cord movement. Chloe's MRI was normal. In other cases, the nerves to the larynx are stretched during a traumatic delivery, particularly when forceps are used. But Chloe was born atraumatically, via cesarean section.

Without a clear cause for her symptoms, the initial approach to Chloe's condition was a period of "watchful waiting" — a medical strategy that involves closely monitoring a patient in hopes of spontaneous improvement without intervention. Chloe remained under observation with a thin nasogastric tube providing her nutrition. When agitated, she often required bag-mask ventilation from her nurse to help her breathe. In cases where there's a reasonable chance of natural resolution, this conservative, wait-and-see approach can be appropriate — as long as the symptoms don't worsen. I decided to give Chloe three weeks to settle. This window allowed time for her young parents to begin processing her condition, while giving the NICU team the opportunity to assess her ongoing stability. The problem with waiting for "spontaneous recovery" with this condition is that it can sometimes take months to years.

The problem with waiting for "spontaneous recovery" with this condition is that it can sometimes take months to years.

Chloe's parents, Cece and Louis, were both just 19 years old and devoutly religious. In the days following her admission, they could always be found praying at her bedside. Meanwhile, fear surrounding the novel coronavirus continued to mount. On March 31, 2020, the first pediatric death from COVID-19 in New York City was recorded. As our hospital began restricting visitors, Cece and Louis were forced to tag-team their daily vigils. Given the NICU's vulnerable population, concern over outside transmission intensifies. Soon, their joint prayer sessions were only condoned via

FaceTime. Despite their unwavering faith, no amount of prayer seemed to resolve Chloe's struggle.

TIME-OUT

This is a 2-week-old full-term healthy infant with biphasic stridor and bilateral vocal-fold immobility, here for a complete airway evaluation.

Chloe's shock of curly red hair garners the attention of the entire OR staff. She has not yet learned to smile, but we all attempt to amuse her anyway. Behind our face shields and N-95 masks, we only have our voices left to comfort these little patients. Chloe is laid down on the operating table. Startled from the transition, she begins crying, which cranks up the volume of her noisy breathing to machine-level. The color in her little pink cheeks begins to drain just as the mask is placed upon her face for pre-oxygenation.

SURGERY START TIME — 7:25 A.M.

Exposing Chloe's airway is easy. She does not have a small jaw, and her mouth opening is wide. There is no sense of immediate urgency. In fact, when sedated, the position of Chloe's relaxed vocal cords actually appears normal.

I use a spatulated instrument to palpate the delicate ball-and-socket joints, to feel the springiness that allows her vocal cords to glide, rotate, or pivot together or apart.

"Cricoarytenoid joints are mobile."

I advance the telescope deeper, entering a wide-open space within a normal caliber airway.

Then, I proceed deeper still until the c-shaped rings of the trachea fork into two main branches, which herald the entrances to the right and left lungs.

"Trachea and airway to carina and first main bronchi are normal. No complete rings, compression, and no malacia (collapse)."

Concluding my evaluation, I turn the operating table back toward anesthesia.

"Her airway is anatomically normal, but sadly, that doesn't solve her problem. Let's wake her up. I need to talk to her parents about their options."

It may come as a surprise, but there is no standard treatment for congenital bilateral vocal-cord paralysis. Management is determined case by case, factoring in the child's anatomy, social circumstances, parental capability, and the skill set of the treating surgeon. Most surgical interventions aim to improve airflow by carving out a controlled opening in the airway to relieve obstruction. This can be achieved through a partial cordotomy (using a laser to notch the vocal cords) or a suture lateralization (pulling one vocal cord open and securing it with a stitch). Another option is an anterior-posterior cricoid split, in which the cricoid cartilage—the ring beneath the vocal cords—is cut and gently pried apart. However, the cartilage tends to spring back closed due to natural tension. To counter this, a balloon is inserted to dilate the area, followed by placement of an oversized endotracheal tube for 5 to 7 days to act as a spacer. This encourages the airway to heal in a widened position with the paralyzed cords slightly open. Alternatively, a synthetic spacer can be used to keep the cricoid ring propped apart.

The final—and most commonly chosen—option is to bypass the problem altogether by placing a tracheostomy tube, giving the child time to grow and potentially regain adductor (opening) function. Though young, Chloe's parents were resolute: they would only consent to a tracheostomy as a last resort, and only after less invasive options were tried and failed.

To be clear, none of the aforementioned procedures can restore the normal physiologic movement of the larynx — its natural opening and closing. Each endoscopic intervention has its own advantages and drawbacks, which we discussed in detail. In cases like this, the typical medical wisdom is to choose the procedure you know best. But with a rare condition like this, few doctors have significant personal experience. We simply don't see enough cases to become truly practiced. I had performed this type of cartilage split only once before — for this exact indication.

In the temporal reality of COVID, I schedule the surgery for the first case, Monday morning.

Although Chloe remains otherwise healthy, Cece becomes acutely symptomatic. She develops high fevers, chills, and then loses her sense of smell. As a known asthmatic, she experiences worsening shortness of breath and requires oxygen and brief hospitalization at a local community hospital. At this point, Louis is no longer allowed to visit his wife or child.

Cece had visited Chloe just two days prior. We convene an internal meeting via Zoom with the parents, NICU, and anesthesia teams to determine the next steps. The NICU decides to place Chloe in isolation to prevent potential spread of COVID-19 to other vulnerable infants. We postpone the surgery for three more days to monitor for symptoms. To everyone's surprise, Chloe never develops any.

TIME-OUT

This is a 4-week-old full-term infant with biphasic stridor and bilateral vocal-fold immobility with no other airway anomalies, who is here for an endoscopic anterior-posterior cricoid split with balloon dilation.

Remember, these were the early days of the pandemic. There was no vaccine. People were dying in staggering numbers across the globe. Every day, I would wake up, turn off my alarm, and check the rising death toll. It was real-life Armageddon and those of us in healthcare were at the epicenter of its fury. We were just as scared for our elderly parents and spouses on immunosuppressants as we were committed to our patients and our Hippocratic duties.

Every day, I would wake up, turn off my alarm, and check the rising death toll. It was real-life Armageddon and those of us in healthcare were at the epicenter of its fury.

SURGERY START TIME — THURSDAY, 8:00 A.M.

There is a palpable tension in the room as I expose Chloe's airway. None of us can help but worry about tiny viral particles lingering in the air, suspended for hours.

I lean forward with my scope and proceed to inject the posterior part of the airway. I position the specialized microscope and focus the larynx under the high-powered lens.

Next, I create a small pocket and carefully separate the fibers of the interarytenoid muscle — a muscle of the larynx that helps close the vocal cords. This maneuver exposes the glistening white surface of the cartilaginous posterior cricoid ring.

"Straight microscissors."

I cut through the cartilage in a sawing motion until I am completely through and through.

"Sickle knife."

I slice through the front portion of the signet-shaped ring with my right hand while palpating the tip of the blade beneath the skin with my left index finger.

The two cartilaginous halves finally spring open.

"7-mm balloon."

"Inflate the balloon up to 14 atmospheres."

The airway widens gradually before our eyes.

"Good. Let's stitch her up. Then, I'll place the tube."

"6.0 dyed Vicryl on a S-14 needle."

"4.5 intubation tube."

The oversized tube passes through the cords with ease. The airway is widened.

"Ok. We're done here. Now we'll see if it's enough for her."

Overall, Chloe's case goes off without a hitch. She remains intubated and sedated for five days, after which the tube is removed as planned. To my delight, in the days following extubation, she thrives. She begins to bottle feed. A bedside scope exam no longer shows a narrow slit — there's now space for her to breathe. It's only about 3 to 4 millimeters, but it's just enough. As per protocol, I schedule her to return to the OR in two weeks for a repeat dilation.

Before that time arrives, Governor Cuomo mandates the cancellation of all non-essential and non-urgent surgeries. The number of coronavirus cases in New York state continues to surge.

Our hospital has become a gloomy place. The infection rates soar. Ventilated patients begin to crowd all empty spaces as their respiratory systems fail. Our bustling children's OR transforms into a ghost town of inactivity. The hospital is on temporary lockdown to any outside transfers. The only sanctioned operative cases are emergencies, trauma, cancer biopsies, and urgent airway cases, like Chloe's.

Another problem arises: a small outbreak among three nurses in Chloe's NICU pod. The timing coincides with her scheduled repeat dilation. This marks the second time our small patient has been exposed to the novel coronavirus. This time, she becomes congested and spikes a fever. Although her oxygen saturation remains stable, she is almost certainly infected.

A heated discussion follows with the Infection Control team. On one hand, we need to contain viral spread within the hospital and avoid unnecessary risk to the operating room team — myself included. On the other, delaying the procedure risks inevitable restenosis of Chloe's airway during this critical window. After extensive deliberation, we decide to proceed — but with strict precautions to limit exposure. No non-essential personnel will be allowed in or out of the OR, including residents, medical students, and circulating nurses. Those in close proximity to Chloe's nose and mouth — namely the anesthesiologist and me — will wear PAPR devices.

PAPR stands for "Powered Air Purifying Respirator," a battery-operated device worn during high-risk, aerosol-generating procedures. It consists of a large white hood with a clear plastic face shield, connected to a waist-mounted fan that draws air through a filter and pushes it into the hood, protecting the wearer from airborne particles.

Laurie, my champion and our OR head nurse, offers to help me suit up — but we both fumble through it. Neither of us has ever used this contraption before. I make sure the breathing tube is attached, and the motor is running, then pull the cover over my head and secure the elastic chin strap. For a moment, I worry about suffocating if something fails. But Laurie double-checks the seal and confirms that the battery pack is fully charged. She gives me a thumbs up. I trust her.

"Tali, you're all good."

Her sweet, singsong voice is partially muted, and her ever-kind smile is hidden behind a duck-like mask — but I can still see the concern in her eyes. Fully geared up, I look like a clone of Dustin Hoffman in the 1990s film *Outbreak*. I'd say it was surreal, but our reality crossed that line long ago — blurred by sirens, lockdowns, mask mandates, and empty grocery shelves.

TIME-OUT

This is a 6.5-week-old full-term infant with congenital bilateral vocal-cord paralysis who is presumably COVID-19 positive and returning to the OR several weeks after an anterior-posterior cricoid split, to repeat the balloon dilation and prevent airway restenosis.

The biggest challenge is the PAPR itself — bulky, with a fan so loud it drowns out the reassuring beep of the monitors. I feel clunky, and communication with my anesthesiologist is limited. Instead of our usual friendly banter, our conversation is purely utilitarian.

"Ok. Let's get started. Get in, dilate, get out."

I'm not convinced that she hears me, but I begin regardless.

SURGERY START TIME — 7:29 A.M.

Throughout the procedure, Chloe's lungs hold relatively steady. Her oxygenation does not drop below the mid-80s, which is abnormal but acceptable. As I begin to inflate the balloon, I can feel the airway stretching beneath me. It hasn't quite clamped back down, but I sense it would have soon.

We did the right thing.

When we are done, Chloe is placed back in her sealed isolette and transported back to her negative-pressure ventilation room in the NICU. She is in stable condition, breathing spontaneously (on her own).

To my relief, she seems even better than before. Her retractions are minimal, and she bottle-feeds with ease. Occasionally, her stridor flares when she's upset, but she continues to breathe comfortably. For the first time, I begin to imagine releasing her into the big, bad world beyond the hospital walls ...

Over the next few weeks — just as I'm signing off on discharge planning — Chloe begins to dwindle. It's not that her noisy breathing has worsened; it hasn't. And it's not because she's sick again — she's tested negative for every virus we can think of. But her oxygen levels are persistently low. Her breathing has grown more rapid and shallow, her nostrils flare even at rest, and the high-pitched stridor has given way to a new, low grunting sound. She starts refusing her bottles entirely, until we have to reinsert the feeding tube. More than once, I find myself simply hovering at her bedside, watching — waiting — worrying.

Chloe's nurse, Sabrina, spots me. Her mama-bear instincts are always on high alert. She and I bonded years ago over another complex-airway baby. Sabrina has dark skin, a brilliant white smile, and wears blue-tinted contacts that turn her brown eyes a mesmerizing shade of violet. It's late in the evening, as we speak quietly under the unit's soft ambient glow. I'm puzzled, trying to make sense of the setback. Chloe's scope exam still looks good. The space between her vocal cords should be enough. So, why isn't it?

It is then that Sabrina casually mentions, "You know she has a murmur, right?"

"No, I didn't."

"She does."

"So, what did cardiology say?"

"Well, she had an echo at the outside hospital when she was born. The transfer note said, 'small PDA.'"

As previously mentioned, a patent ductus arteriosus (PDA) is a heart defect where a blood vessel called the ductus arteriosus, which normally closes shortly after birth, remains open. This common finding is rarely relevant to an airway problem. In this particular case, it became important.

"Has it closed?"

"I don't know … They said it was, 'likely to resolve spontaneously.'"

I borrow her stethoscope and place the small round bell against Chloe's sinking chest. I hear a continuous whooshing sound.

"I'm no cardiologist, but that's pretty audible. Maybe her problem is no longer her airway. Maybe it's her heart."

"I don't know, Doc ... maybe it is."

When I first push for a cardiac reevaluation, I'm met with the usual resistance. And I get it — everyone in the hospital is stretched thin, overworked, and understaffed. Many cardiologists have already been redeployed to help manage the mounting ICU burden. Consultations for viral-induced myocarditis are at an all-time high. So, at first, my concerns are dismissed.

"It must be the airway. It's unlikely the heart."

Still, I do not relent. To be honest, I rarely do. Partly due to my tenacity, and partly because of her obviously worsening condition, a repeat echocardiogram is finally performed. It reveals a significant decline in Chloe's heart function, caused by a large shunt—an abnormal flow of blood—that's overloading her lungs and placing increased strain on her heart.

Still, I do not relent. To be honest, I rarely do.

The very next day, Chloe is taken to the operating room by the head of pediatric cardiothoracic surgery for open-heart surgery to close her patent ductus arteriosus.

Although I do not speak to the surgeon directly, per report (from a scrub nurse I spoke to), he comments intraoperatively, "Wow, that is one *hugely* dilated vessel."

True to her fiery red hair, Chloe proves once again that she's a fighter. Her recovery is swift and successful. Her breathing, once visibly labored, becomes almost effortless. She eats, sleeps, and cries without danger — just as an infant should. Her vocal cords still don't open properly, but for now, she can breathe.

Finally, her entire care team agrees that it is time to release her to home. And although nervous in the pits of our stomachs … we do.

DEBRIEF

"Just because you are a hammer (or pediatric otolaryngologist) doesn't mean everything is a nail."

"Avoid tunnel vision. Think outside the box. If it's not the airway, don't forget the heart, the lungs and the brain."

"Never be reflexively dismissive … because you will be wrong at least half of the time."

"When consulting in the NICU, remember to talk to the nurses. They are the watchdogs for these little humans, constantly fighting to keep them alive. Just assume they know much more than you do."

"Sometimes there is much to be gained by just listening to those around you."

"Pursue all avenues when a patient is declining. Better to hit a few dead ends than to never find the right path forward."

"Be mindfully courageous when need be. Stay safe but still be willing to push yourself to the limit of your skillset to help your patient."

"When the world shuts down (and, due to COVID-19, it has in our lifetime), you may find yourself to be their only hope."

AT HOME

Chloe was born while the world outside her was imploding. Normal life had ground to a screeching halt, the economy teetered on collapse, and society was ordered to shelter in place. Still, we doctors and nurses had a job to do. Every day, we ventured out into danger. Our mudrooms became decontamination zones. We accepted the risk — always with the gnawing fear of bringing the virus home to those we loved. Behind the scenes of our professional lives, our personal lives were unraveling too. Schools shut down, and all in-person learning came to an abrupt end.

Normal life had ground to a screeching halt, the economy teetered on collapse, and society was ordered to shelter in place. Still, we doctors and nurses had a job to do. Every day, we ventured out into danger.

The impact of this shift was different for each of my children. For my oldest daughter, it was surprisingly positive. Freed from the peer pressures and organizational demands of school, she began to blossom. My middle daughter, on the other hand, grew miserable. She deeply missed the social connection of her friend group and cursed the "glitchy" frustration of online learning. For my youngest, who relied on various in-school support services, remote learning was an outright disaster. Without constant redirection, she couldn't stay focused, and in the absence of a structured environment and trained educators, she floundered.

My husband, like many others, was holed up in a makeshift attic office (he's a senior IT project manager). Though he was already somewhat accustomed to remote work — standard in the tech world — the prolonged isolation and the total lack of face-to-face interactions wore on him. Similarly, the effect of prolonged isolation cut just as deep.

As for me, the initial six weeks of the COVID shutdown offered me the longest relative break of my entire adult life (including maternity leave with each of my three children). With elective surgeries and office-based medicine paused, my daily grind abated. Our department remained responsible for otolaryngologic emergencies, managed through an on-call system. For high-risk cases — like adult tracheostomies on floridly COVID-positive patients — special protocols were developed. We rotated coverage to evenly distribute the exposure risk among us. And yet, despite the high-stakes hospital obligations, there was downtime. During that brief, less-than-two-month window, I was able to be physically and emotionally present in ways I never had been before.

My long-dormant creative side was finally allowed to flourish. I started — and actually finished — house projects. My favorite accomplishment was transforming our living room into a calm oasis of zen. Using soothing greens and muted pinks, I decorated the space with my dream chinoiserie wallpaper — an intricate pattern of birds and trees that I discovered after endless scrolling on Etsy. I also curated my first-ever photo gallery in the upstairs hallway, featuring some of my most treasured images of my father, who I still achingly missed *every single day*.

On several mornings, I sat next to Alex on the stone front porch, coffee in hand. I even ate breakfast — a weekday luxury only reserved for people with time, something I never seemed to have. Like many hunkered-down families, we welcomed our first dog: Junie, the most smoochable, precious Goldendoodle, who brought more love into our lives than I ever could have imagined. My sweet girls formed an unshakable bond — one forged through excessive time together, shared loneliness, and separation from their peers. Even my 72-year-old mother found renewed closeness in a lifelong, complicated relationship with her 75-year-old sister, after the two were unexpectedly stranded together in Deerfield Beach, Florida, for months at the start of the pandemic.

Amid immense human suffering, a few rays of light managed to pierce through. As "first responders," we were momentarily elevated — basking in a wave of societal appreciation. Our personal sacrifices were recognized, even admired. Each time I drove down the hospital road, my eyes met a line of banners reading, "Heroes work here." Of course, whatever small silver linings emerged, I would never have wished this plague upon our planet. The global loss of life, the long-term health consequences, and the devastating effects of long-COVID far outweighed any collateral benefits. Like everyone around me, I prayed for stability — and celebrated the long-awaited development of a vaccine.

In December 2020, the first COVID-19 vaccines in the United States were administered to hospital personnel. It marked the beginning of our slow return to normalcy. Full recovery would take years, but at last, we had a start. Finally, there was hope.

CHAPTER 15

BLACK CLOUDS AND AWAKE TRACHS

THE "BLACK CLOUD" phenomenon in medicine refers to the superstitious belief that certain individuals — residents or attendings — attract an unusually high volume of admissions or difficult cases. It's widely accepted in healthcare culture, even without scientific proof. We believe in it because, frankly, we've lived it. Studies have tried to determine whether there's any truth to it — maybe it's not just spirits and voodoo, but a reflection of personal or hospital-specific factors. Whatever the explanation, whenever my senior resident, Annie, and I are on call together, I sleep in my scrubs. We cover all ages at the hospital for ENT problems. So, when she rings me at 10:00 p.m. on a Friday night, I'm not surprised by the urgency in her voice. The moment I saw our names side by side on the call schedule, I knew the storm was coming.

"Hi. I just saw a 60-something-year-old woman BIBA (brought-in-by-ambulance) for increased work of breathing and disorientation. She has a past history of total thyroidectomy and post-op radiation for thyroid cancer with resulting bilateral vocal-cord paralysis. She previously had a tracheostomy, which supposedly was removed at the outside facility last year."

Annie sends me a video over TigerText, our secure hospital messaging system. The patient's vocal cords are barely opening, and the diameter of the airway is miniscule. Not good. Not good at all.

> *"I think she's gonna need an awake trach."*

> *"Book it."*

An "awake trach" refers to a tracheostomy performed while the patient is awake rather than under full anesthesia. Local anesthetic is injected into the neck to numb the area, but the patient continues to breathe spontaneously as the surgical team creates the opening to secure the airway. This approach is typically used in cases of severe upper airway obstruction, where intubation from above isn't possible. It's a method of stabilizing the airway when time is of the essence and general anesthesia is simply too risky.

By the time I reach the holding area, the patient, Gloria, is too confused to give consent. She is maintaining her saturation with supplemental oxygen, but she's tiring out. She is mouthing something I can only deduce is, "my son, my son."

I call the number on the chart for her son, Phillip, who lives five hours away in Burlington, Vermont.

"Hello, this is Dr. Lando. I am the ENT surgeon on call. Your mother, Gloria, was brought into the hospital in severe respiratory distress. We need to secure her airway immediately. You are listed as her healthcare proxy. Will you give your consent for us to perform an emergency tracheostomy?"

"But I just visited her last week, and she was fine. What happened?"

"I don't know but we need to focus on helping her right now. Do I have your permission to proceed?"

"Yes, Doc. Do whatever she needs."

Time-Out

This is a 67-year-old female in extremis, here for an awake trach. The fire risk is high, but the oxygen will be lowered to room air right before we enter the airway.

The patient's airway is so precarious that we can't lay her flat for optimal positioning. The anesthesiologist is uncomfortable sedating her, fearing any suppression of her natural respiratory drive. After we prep, Annie injects local anesthetic into the skin, and the patient reacts more than I'd like. We expect this to be an easy chip shot — she already has a clear indentation marking the previous surgical site.

Pop in, stabilize, get out, get home.

Surgery Start Time — 11:45 p.m.

I grab the 15-blade scalpel in my right hand and proceed. After some spreading, I see the telltale bubbling of secretions, indicating entry into the airway. But the anatomy is distorted. Despite the lidocaine, the patient is so intolerant of the pressure that she bucks straight upward, nearly levitating off the operating table.

Bloody mucous splatters across our face shields. Despite the mess, we continue working to widen the entry hole. I angle the tracheostomy tube as usual.

Ninety degrees, insert, then rotate.

The tube doesn't go in as easily as usual. The oxygen levels rise, but only to the low 90s. When the ventilator begins delivering respirations, the patient's neck and face start to swell. I palpate the neck and feel the unmistakable crinkly tell-tell sign of crepitus.

Shit.

Subcutaneous emphysema — also known as crepitus — is a sign that air has dissected through the tissue planes beneath the skin. In this case, it suggests a tear in the trachea. We suspect that her forceful bucking, combined with a history of prior radiation to the neck and chest, may have weakened the tracheal wall. Despite this concern, she's maintaining decent air exchange … until suddenly, she isn't.

"I've lost CO2."

I re-adjust the trach tube, applying upward pressure.

"Got it back."

I relax my grip.

"What about now?"

"Gone again. Sats dropping … 85 … 75 …"

"Hand me the 5.0 fiberoptic GlideScope."

The GlideScope is an airway visualization system, which projects onto a portable screen.

I quickly guide the long white rubber flexible scope through the tube, hoping to see the pink-walled branches of the bronchi leading toward the right and left lungs. Instead, I just see a bizarre dark space with scattered fronds of yellow tissue.

"What on earth are we looking at?" the anesthesiologist asks, perplexed.

"Damn it. It's the party wall."

The "party wall" between the trachea and the esophagus refers to the shared membranous wall at the posterior aspect of the trachea. It separates the trachea (airway) from the esophagus (digestive tract). It is made up of fibroelastic membranes and rare muscle fibers. That's *not* where I should be.

I pull the tube back ever so slightly and the view becomes recognizable.

"Now, I'm in the airway."

Despite the troubling findings, the patient remains stable — for now. But the situation is too precarious. I make the call.

"Janine, I need your help."

I quickly elucidate the facts.

"Janine, are you there?"

"Yes," she whispers. "I've just put the baby down."

If I had more time, I could call around to Mike Y. or Steve H. or Dave G. Any one of them would willingly drive in to help. But there isn't any time.

"I'm so sorry. I still need you. Can you come?"

She pauses, but I know her. She'll always do the right thing. Sometimes, it just takes a minute to process the unexpected disruption.

"Ok. I'll be there. Will take a bit, though."

"Thank you. We'll be waiting."

Dr. Janine Rotsides is our younger head-and-neck reconstructive surgeon. Just back from maternity leave, she is still adjusting to the intensity of working life as a new mom with a nanny. I get it. I've been there — three times around.

It feels like an eternity until she arrives in the room, but luckily the patient's vitals have been holding steady.

Janine scrubs in, and Annie instinctively steps aside. She widens the incision, then begins methodically probing the area, assessing the damage. We already know there's a rent somewhere. It isn't immediate — but eventually, she finds the source.

"I think we just need a longer tube. We should be ok. Within a week, the airway should seal up on its own."

We replace the standard tube with an XLT (extra-long tracheostomy tube).

The saturation rises to 98% and doesn't fluctuate.

"You good?"

"I'm good."

"OK. I'm gonna head out and try to catch the baby's next bottle."

"I really appreciate the help. You're the best ... really."

"No problem."

I feel guilty to have pulled her in, but am deeply appreciative, nonetheless.

We're all in the same crazy circus, constantly juggling ... family-work, work-family.

Annie and I finish up. Gloria's body will gradually reabsorb the trapped air.

I step out to call her son with an update. He's on the way, still driving.

"Your mom is okay. The new tracheostomy tube is in place. There were some difficulties with the placement, so just be prepared — she's going to look extremely swollen. It may be a bit shocking at first, but it will get better. We'll begin trying to wean her from the ventilator over the next few days."

LATER

Even in a busy hospital like ours, the odds of two airway emergencies in one weekend are very slim. Most of the time, months pass without a single emergency "awake trach" on our department's watch. So, with one case already behind me, I'm feeling pretty relaxed as I slip into my grey and white pinstripe pajamas on Sunday at 10:00 p.m. My Monday OR schedule is packed — tight as sardines. I plug in my phone, ready to let it charge overnight. I even risk setting my alarm for 6:15 a.m. the next morning. So, inevitably … beep, beep, beep …

> *Dr. Lando, I'm so sorry to bother you, but it's urgent. We have another one.*

Damn it. Seriously?

Fifty-two minutes and forty-seven seconds later …

TIME-OUT (TAKE TWO)

This is a 55-year-old unvaccinated male, recently emigrated from Guatemala, who presents with diffuse swelling of the supraglottic tissues. He arrived at our ED an hour ago with his wife, unable to speak clearly or swallow his secretions. His scope exam revealed diffuse swelling with a barely identifiable pinpoint airway.

I do not believe he can be tubed from above. He is here for an awake tracheostomy.

At least this time, the patient isn't thrashing on the OR table. His muscles are tense, neck vessels bulging. He's clearly terrified — but he's listening intently.

Hey, Siri … translate to Spanish, "You need to remain perfectly still."

"Necesitas permanecer perfectamente quieto."

"You may feel pressure in your neck, but DO NOT MOVE."

"Puede que sientas presión en el cuello, pero NO TE MUEVAS."

Adult supraglottitis is a potentially life-threatening condition marked by inflammation of the laryngeal structures above the vocal cords. Patients can rapidly develop airway compromise, which may lead to respiratory arrest. While usually caused by bacterial or viral infections, supraglottitis can also result from non-infectious sources, such as inflammatory reaction or thermal injury.

In less technical terms, it's serious. You gotta move fast and establish a safe airway, quickly.

"Knife … suction … retractors … cric hook … scissors … dilator … trach tube …."

"Do we have CO_2?"

"Yes."

This time around, the case is straightforward and trouble-free. It goes off without a hitch.

Once the trach is in, the patient's distress abruptly abates. Though he still can't talk, he can now breathe.

The good news is he should do well once the swelling resolves. It may take a few days but, hopefully, we can decannulate him (remove the trach tube) prior to discharge.

It's past midnight.

All I can think is: thank G-d for small favors. I'm not sure I could stomach calling Janine again this weekend.

Then, I remember the time-tested adage … bad things in our hospital always come in threes!

DEBRIEF

"Not all things go well all the time. Actually, assume they might not. Have contingency plans A and B and even C."

"Sometimes we're forced to deal with suboptimal circumstances. It may be due to intrinsic patient characteristics or extrinsic factors or both. The key is in recognizing the problem and adjusting the plan, even when all you want to do is freak the hell out."

"Remember your lifelines. Don't hesitate to 'phone a friend,' if needed. You might feel embarrassed — but don't be. The best outcome is always worth it."

"Accept help but always pay it forward. Say 'yes' to your colleagues when you can — even when the timing is inconvenient."

"If you do lend a hand, do it out of selflessness — not for praise, payback, or recognition."

"Remember it's the patient receiving the favor, so don't make your colleagues feel guilty about it later."

Last, but not least …

"You can't escape the black-cloud resident — hell, they might be your favorite. So, suit up for the storm like a pro. When on call, don't ditch your scrubs like I did."

AT HOME

I don't want to leave the impression that my work/life balance is all #SuperMom — it's not. At home, I'm often cranky and overtired. I rarely cook (unless reheating leftovers or boiling Wacky Mac counts), and I loathe cleaning, despite wanting my house to look like a spotless oasis. Most days, I burn through all my patience at work and have nothing left for reviewing test material about the American Revolution — or helping with math homework, especially.

I don't want to leave the impression that my work/life balance is all #SuperMom — it's not.

I don't recommend trying to do it all — no one can. My motto is actually: "Outsource whatever possible." These days, Alex handles most of the shuttling to games and activities. Frankly, even before him, it was never me. It was a rotating cast of wonderful young Brazilian au pairs and, before that, a lineup of nannies of all ages. In recent years, I've upped our housekeeper, Dione, to three days a week just to maintain basic cleanliness and preserve my sanity. Still, my kitchen is always an inexplicable mess.

Over time, my older kids have gotten skilled at reading my moods and adjusting their requests accordingly. When I'm clearly overwhelmed, they're amazingly mature and helpful. Still, despite my predictably snippy reactions, Milla never fails to ask, "Mommy, why do you always come home so annoyed?"

When I'm home, but on call, it's definitely worse for them. My acid reflux flares from the constant interruptions, texts, and calls. Like most doctors, I hate the tease of being "off of the clock" while feeling the tension of having to return at a moment's notice.

As expected, after my patients and my kids, Alex gets the dregs of me. If I'm not demanding and short-tempered, then I'm usually lethargic and distracted. The common refrain, "Do you mind if we talk about it later?" stands in for the never uttered but highly coveted, "What did *you* want to talk about, honey?" Even when I make a concerted effort not to bring my work home, I always do. This is both physically — in the form of countless unwritten notes — and mentally, in every possible way.

When I ask, "What did you say?" Alex often replies (less of a complaint than an observation), "Forget it. I know I'm just the white noise in the background."

Even when I'm off the clock, my mind is often adrift. Even when I'm truly off-off, it takes a minimum of three days of vacation for me to relax and reset. At this point, it's usually about time to go home. Back at work, it takes the same amount of time to get back in the zone, making the time off feel pointless.

You may now want to ask, "Knowing all this, would you make the same choices again?"

For me, the answer is simple. Even after all these years — despite the exhaustion, the sacrifices, and the disheartening ways in which medicine has evolved — I wouldn't trade it for anything. Not for anything at all.

A BIT OF PERSPECTIVE

Any way you slice it, this profession is hard. The hospital environment is tough. Surgery can be physically and mentally grueling. The commitment is lifelong. For those who choose a career in medicine — especially those who choose to go into surgery — there will be countless forces beating you down. So, find the ones that lift you up. There will be low points, epic saves, and cataclysmic losses. Not everyone will love you. In fact, many won't. I can't promise it will ever be easy.

Any way you slice it, this profession is hard.
The hospital environment is tough. Surgery can
be physically and mentally grueling.
The commitment is lifelong.

But if you're really and truly lucky, you can be a person who gets to wake up every single morning with a clear sense of purpose, just like me.

DIAGRAM OF
THE SINUS ANATOMY

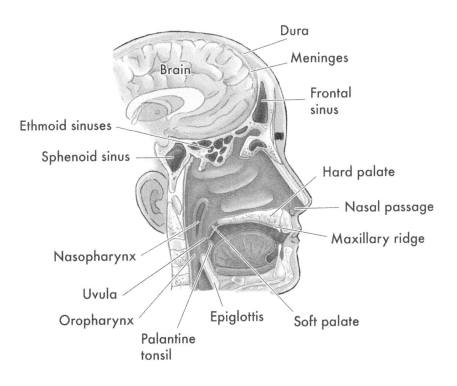

Dura

Meninges

Brain

Frontal sinus

Ethmoid sinuses

Sphenoid sinus

Hard palate

Nasal passage

Maxillary ridge

Nasopharynx

Uvula

Oropharynx

Epiglottis

Soft palate

Palantine tonsil

Illustration by Juliette Aronoff

CHAPTER 16

"IT MUST BE LOVE (PUS) ON THE BRAIN"

MOST PEOPLE THINK sinus infections are limited to those pesky bouts of congestion, slime-green phlegm, and a hacking cough. But few realize they can lead to shockingly serious complications. In a large medical center, we sometimes see sinus infections that are life-threatening. Often, by the time these patients reach us, they've already suffered a major neurologic injury. To understand why, you need a basic sense of the anatomy.

The sinuses are air-filled cavities that help humidify inhaled air, lighten the skull, and trap dirt, dust, and pollutants by producing mucus. These paired chambers are in the cheeks (maxillary), between the eyes (ethmoid), in the forehead (frontal), and deep within the skull (sphenoid). The trouble begins when infection breaches the bony walls surrounding them, putting nearby critical structures — like the brain and eyes — at risk. Infection can also travel through veins or arteries, spreading into the bloodstream or forming septic emboli — infectious clots that block blood flow and cause strokes. The escalation from "I have a bad sinus headache" to "I can't see in my right eye" can be astonishingly fast. The added danger in my patient population — young children — is that they may not articulate anything at all … until the severity of their situation can no longer be ignored … until the damage is already done.

My Friday clinics are supercharged, always busy and then packed to the gills with "can you just see them before the weekend" add-ons from colleagues and referring pediatricians. I scurry between my three patient rooms like a squirrrel late to a nut sale. Routine follow-ups for ear tubes and tonsillectomies are often mixed with complex tracheostomy cases — kids with obscure syndromes and layered medical histories. On this particular Friday, I am 85% done with patients (only 30% done with paperwork), running on one Diet Coke, one latte, and fumes. It's been a hectic week — made worse by the start of my first weekend call of the new year, which kicked off hours before the last patient even left the waiting room.

The moment the clock strikes five, my hospital text pings. I've just finished explaining the details of a necessary endoscopic airway surgery to a pair of emotional first-time parents.

Dr. Lando. Please call me.

"Excuse me. I have to take this. It's the hospital."

I step into the hallway.

"Katherine, what's up?"

"We just got a consult about a teenager being brought in from a nearby hospital with suspected meningitis and cranial neuropathies. I already ordered an emergency CT sinuses with stealth."

"Ok, lemme know when you have an update."

"Will do."

Evelyn is a bright 18-year-old college sophomore studying electrical engineering. Ten days before her transfer to our hospital, she contracted adenovirus — the common cold. Over the next several days, she developed headaches, nausea, high fevers, and mild neck pain. When her symptoms worsened, she visited an urgent care clinic near her college and was prescribed an oral antibiotic. The following morning, she woke up confused. Her roommate then saw her eyes roll back, her face droop on the right, and her speech become slurred. Moments later, Evelyn collapsed in a full-body seizure. When the ambulance arrived, she was unresponsive but still breathing. She was intubated on site and brought to a local hospital, where initial brain imaging showed abnormalities in both the language and motor centers. Plans were made for immediate helicopter transfer to our medical center, but high winds and fog grounded the flight. Instead, Evelyn endured a six-hour ambulance ride to reach us.

Upon arrival, Evelyn only opens her eyes to stimulation. She can't respond to questions or follow commands. Her parents, visibly overwhelmed, crouch at her bedside — having raced in from their suburban home. Her mother reports that Evelyn has no history of sinus infections, immune deficiencies, or any family history of autoimmune or blood disorders. A comprehensive battery of tests is ordered: bloodwork to assess for clotting problems, a more detailed MRI of the brain, a CT scan of the sinuses, and a CT angiogram to evaluate the surrounding blood vessels.

By the time I finish with my last patient of the day, Katherine texts me.

> The imaging is loaded into PACs.
> Does not look good.

Evelyn's MRI reveals extensive abnormal enhancement of the meninges — the brain's protective lining — suggestive of widespread inflammation.

The CT angiogram — with its tree-like vessels branching in all directions — reveals critical narrowing of both internal carotid arteries. These arteries supply the brain with blood and oxygen and pass through hollow structures called the cavernous sinuses, which also house vital nerves responsible for vision, eye movement, and facial sensation. An infection in the nearby sphenoid sinuses can trigger a chain reaction: it spreads to the arterial walls, incites inflammation, and leads to the formation of infected clots (thrombi). These clots can break off, travel through the bloodstream, and block smaller vessels (septic emboli), cutting off blood flow and triggering neurologic symptoms. I study the squiggles on my screen — segments of Evelyn's carotid arteries appear narrowed and irregular.

The CT of the sinuses elucidates the origin of this terrible cascade. Evelyn's sphenoid sinuses — normally air-filled and outlined by white bone — are completely opacified, appearing gray, a sign they're filled with fluid or infected tissue. This suggests a significant nidus of infection. Given the severity of her neurologic symptoms, this is now an urgent case of pus under pressure near the brain. The infection must be drained as expeditiously as possible.

My busy day is about to get much longer.
I text Katherine.

> Book it now.

The OR is readied, and the ENT Stealth machine is wheeled in. This technology provides real-time, 3D-image guidance during surgery, allowing us to navigate delicate sinus anatomy in real-time with precision — avoiding critical structures like the optic nerves and skull base.

All the instrument trays are lined up and opened. The relevant instruments are laid out.

Two screens are arranged side-by-side at eye-level — endoscopic view to the right, CT image guidance to the left, by convention.

TIME-OUT

This is an 18-year-old previously healthy college student with multiple neurologic deficits resulting from acute sphenoid sinusitis and secondary carotid artery stenosis with septic emboli. The plan for today is to open and drain the sphenoid sinuses and obtain cultures.

Evelyn has been extubated since soon after her arrival. Her breathing is not labored. She is surprisingly calm, looking out from her stretcher with an expressionless gaze. When touched, she retracts asymmetrically, her right arm pulling away as her left-sided limbs stay limp at her side, barely moving from their place.

Evelyn is positioned on the table, her head cushioned by a thick gel mattress. Beneath it, the electromagnetic emitter plate is carefully angled. The image-guided instruments are calibrated to within 1 mm of precision. Each tool is registered: straight probe, fine suction, gently curved 90-degree suctions. Her nasal cavity is decongested.

Surgery Start Time — 7:55 p.m.

The telescope is gently inserted into the nose, projecting the image onto the overhead screen. There's work to be done before we reach our destination. Some structures must be lateralized (pushed to the side), others reflected (flipped up), and still others — bone and mucosal lining alike — must be opened, chipped, or chomped away. The targets, the sphenoid sinuses, lie deep in the center of the cranial cavity. Endoscopic surgery in this region demands precise identification of anatomical landmarks and careful orientation within the surgical field to avoid complications.

There are two main ways to approach the sphenoid sinuses. One is an anterior-to-posterior route, working through the closest sinus cells and gradually progressing deeper. The other is a more direct method — the paraseptal approach — which targets the sphenoids right through the middle of the nose with less disruption to surrounding tissue. This is the route we choose for Evelyn. The goal is clear: release the dangerous infection and get her safely off the table.

The heart-rate monitor pitch rises rapidly in response to the placement of cotton pledgets soaked in epinephrine to decongest her nose and improve visibility.

I glance up from the screen to my anesthesiologist, eyebrows raised.

"She's ok. Strong young heart."

More than any other sinus, the sphenoid is boxed in. The challenge lies in its highly variable size and location. Go too high and you can penetrate the brain or cause a cerebrospinal fluid (CSF) leak. Go too lateral and you risk optic nerve trauma, or major bleeding caused by an internal carotid artery injury. It's a tight, high-stakes space, so the key is to be methodical.

I push the middle turbinate out of the way with a slim metal instrument called a Freer elevator. The nasal septum curves slightly medial. I advance the scope into the tight space between them. The superior turbinate comes clearly into view.

"There it is. Straight through-cut please."

"Upbiting Kerrison."

"J-curette."

"There's the sphenoid opening."

I move the probe slightly up and medial to find the point of least resistance and ... pop!

Bright yellow pus spills forth, filling the screen.

G-d. It's just soooo satisfying.

"Culture swab. Suction."

"Small mushroom punch to widen the opening."

More gooey purulent material cascades over the edge of the new opening.

"Warm saline irrigation in a bulb syringe. Keep it coming."

"Ok, team. That's great. Let's start wrapping it up."

Evelyn is awoken from anesthesia for transport back to the ICU in stable condition. She opens her eyes briefly, then drifts back to sleep.

Our work is done for tonight, but the impact of her illness is far from over.

Over the next few days, Evelyn's fevers do subside. She becomes more alert, and her face begins to move more symmetrically. But still she says nothing.

"When will she talk?" her parents ask in desperation.

Evelyn's initial MRI showed signs of evolving infection and swelling, but no clear infarct (stroke) or evidence of acute blood deprivation to the brain. This is encouraging. Some of her early lab results point to a possible underlying disorder, which may explain why the infection progressed so aggressively despite an otherwise normal immune system.

"We don't know. Her brain took a big hit. There is so much inflammation. She needs time."

"How much time?"

I have no concrete answers. The neurologist will weigh in, but he, too, will have no clarity.

Over the next week, Evelyn begins to show slow but meaningful signs of improvement. Her vacant stare gives way to a clearer attentiveness. She starts moving her left arm and leg, albeit hesitantly. With the help of a physical therapist, she even begins to bear weight. Still, she remains mute.

On day 10, despite broad-spectrum antibiotics and our successful drainage of the inciting infection in her sinuses, Evelyn experiences a noticeable decline. She becomes withdrawn and groggy. Her eager eyes glaze over. She develops a left facial droop, her fevers return, and she develops a pounding headache, which she signals by covering her forehead. An urgent repeat MRI is obtained, and another dreaded complication becomes a reality. The MRI reveals extension of the infection beneath the dura, or outermost layer of the brain, through the sphenoid bone into the part of the skull base that houses the frontal lobes of the brain. There is swelling in both lobes, or cerebritis.

Skull-base infections have significant morbidity and mortality, requiring prompt and aggressive management. When necessary, surgery to drain these subdural empyemas (collections of pus beneath the lining of the brain) is performed by neurosurgery. This is an example of where two specialties both intersect and complement each other. While the neurosurgeon retains domain in the brain, a fellowship-trained ENT skull-base surgeon (not me) is often involved in the approach, helping to gain endoscopic access to the area. Luckily, there are several excellent super-specialists in our hospital.

At this point, I could instruct the primary team to page neurosurgery—but that has to run up the chain of command, and delays are common. I could tell my resident to call our skull-base surgeon directly, but that might not convey the urgency. I could take a passive role—after all, it's not exactly my place to push others to intervene. I could give instructions, walk away, go home, and hear about it later.

But none of those are the things I do.

Instead, I stay involved. I text selected MRI slices, a summary of the relevant history, and the key lab and culture results to a group chat with our rhinology/skull-base surgeons, Drs. Ashleigh Halderman and Patricia Johnson — and Avi, one of the many wonderful pediatric neurosurgeons, Dr. Avinash Mohan (along with Drs. Carrie Muh, Jared Pisapia, and Michael Tobias). Once the message is delivered and read, I call each of them directly, then merge the calls, forcing an immediate meeting of the minds between the two services. I stay on the line, on mute, listening in the background as they review the scans and formulate a collaborative plan.

After all that, it's my time to pass the baton.

CONTINUATION AND THE RED-CARPET CEREMONY

I won't get into the details of Evelyn's second surgery because I didn't perform it, and because I wasn't present for its entirety. What I will say is that it was both technically demanding and remarkably successful. Despite the risks, the infection was fully drained, with no complications and no significant blood loss (kudos to those involved).

Initially, Evelyn remains in the ICU, but once she stabilizes, she is transferred to the standard unit. With the help of multiple culture-directed antibiotics — guided by the Infectious Disease team — along with steroids and blood thinners, she slowly but steadily improves again. To her parents' delight, she begins to speak; after weeks of silence, Evelyn starts responding with simple "yes" or "no" answers. Over the course of time, those brief responses evolve into intelligible phrases.

After a month and a half in the hospital, she is finally ready for discharge. Sadly, she's not yet ready to return home — but she will leave for an intensive physical and neurologic rehabilitation center.

The red-carpet ceremony is a special tradition at our children's hospital, reserved for patients who have endured life-threatening illnesses or injuries and prolonged hospital stays. It's a big deal. For Evelyn, it marks the culmination of a long journey: 25 grueling days in intensive care, followed by 20 more on the pediatric floor.

In preparation for the fête, a wide red carpet is rolled out — from her hospital room all the way to the exit sign. When the announcement booms over the PA system, people begin to gather. Soon, the hallways are lined on both sides with hospital staff: doctors and nurses, social workers and unit clerks, security officers and cleaning personnel — all converging to honor her.

It's one of those rare, unifying moments you don't want to miss. Sure, it's a little cheesy — but it's also undeniably uplifting: a celebration of life, human resilience, and the power of teamwork and modern medicine.

Evelyn's entire family is there — people of all ages: aunts, uncles, cousins, and of course, her parents. Even her dad's old college fraternity buddies have traveled down to show their support. "Live Your Life," Evelyn's favorite Rihanna song, pumps through the portable speaker system. The Child Life Specialists pass around maracas and tambourines, urging everyone to shake and rattle in anticipation of her appearance.

The air is vibrating with emotion. When Evelyn finally emerges from her room, she looks around at the crowd — and is overcome with emotion. We erupt in cheers as the EMT pushes her elevated stretcher down the long red carpet. More people file in, clapping, whistling, whooping, and calling out messages of strength and congratulations.

There isn't a dry eye in the place.

So live your life (hey, ayy, ayy, ayy)
You steady chasin' that paper, just live your life
(Oh, ayy ayy ayy)
Ain't got no time for no haters, just live your life
(Hey, ayy ayy ayy)
No tellin' where it'll take ya, just live your life

As Evelyn and her parents reach the exit sign, the elevator dings. Soon, they are almost out of sight.

Then, right before the metal doors slide close, her dad turns back and catches my tear-stained eye.

He mouths, "Thank you."

LATER

For patients with neurologic injury, the battle never ends within the hospital walls. If anything, their challenges have just begun. These patients now face the impossible task of returning to a familiar life with an entirely different reality. Tasks that used to be as natural as walking and talking may need to be relearned. Muscles — once strong and lean but now weak with disuse — must be retrained. With each incremental step forward, there are countless new benchmarks to achieve.

At her first post-op visit, I am astonished by Evelyn's progress. She is communicative. Her responses are terse but appropriate. She is walking independently, she's engaged, and she's actually smiling, at times. Despite my delight at her improvement, she is frustrated with the pace. Previously an excellent student and easy conversationalist, she now struggles with reading and with verbal fluency. Her memory is faulty, and information slips out soon after entry leaving little solidly retained. Math concepts, once so obvious even in their obscurity, elude her on a very basic level.

In general, the good news is that neural plasticity in children is robust, which means that their brains have a greater ability to recover lost function and reorganize. Pediatric brains are still developing and have a larger supply of available neural connections; these connections can be recruited to take over for areas damaged by stroke, infection, or injury. The functional outcomes for young patients like Evelyn can often surpass those of older patients facing similar medical crises. At 18, Evelyn occupies a "middle ground" between adolescence and adulthood — her brain still retains a greater capacity for remodeling and recovery, provided she receives appropriate rehabilitation.

Still, she will need time, effort, and a great deal of patience. Even then, her new "normal" is unlikely to fully resemble what it once was.

Evelyn's next several follow-up visits are more social than medical. I'm elated to see her back at school — albeit with a limited course load and various accommodations. I take extra time to tell her how impressed I am with her determination and resilience. It's all true, and it never hurts to hear that again and again.

"Evelyn, you are a superhero. Never forget that. I am in awe of how far you've come, and I am lucky to know you. I am so proud to have been even a small part of your amazing story."

DEBRIEF

"Know when to act with urgency, even if a patient problem has been brewing for days."

"Go with your gut when your gut says time is of the essence. It probably is."

"Sure, the cat may already be out of the bag (e.g., the infection may already be widespread), but you can never know when the impact on the patient will reach the point of no return (in this case, complete neurologic devastation). Do something when you can."

"There will be instances when you must convince your colleagues to get involved and take immediate action. Though you may feel it is not your job, do it anyway."

"You may find yourself doing tasks that are 'beneath you.' They are not. You are doing it for the patient. Feel proud. You care that much."

"There are times you will be perceived as pushy, 'super annoying,' even an 'alarmist.' Be ok with those monikers. Don't back down. In the end, it's worth it. Your patients will benefit."

"It's okay to get personal, to encourage your patients — even when your advice goes beyond the strict boundaries of your specialty. It's good to give a little extra of yourself and your soul."

"You will not lose anything. You may actually find something inside yourself."

"It may feel like a reach, but your patients will know you truly care — and they'll appreciate it more than you can imagine."

AT HOME

Life outside the hospital can be messy and complicated. Inside my OR, the priorities are so clear. Focus on the patient, fix the patient. Orient the room, white-balance the camera, calibrate the navigation system. Place the speculum in the nares (nostrils), insert the pledgets, look inside. Identify the landmarks and begin. The necessary equipment is all there. The instruments are ready. Just follow the steps. Open the sinuses, drain the pus. Adrenaline is pumping through my body, overcoming the exhaustion.

Life outside the hospital can be messy and complicated. Inside my OR, the priorities are so clear.

When the wind blasts my face as I finally step outside, my sails often deflate. A flood of realizations washes over me, reminding me of all the loose ends I left untied at home. The oven is broken, and I forgot to purchase the extended warranty ... or maybe I did but I misplaced the receipt. I missed the early deadline to sign the kids up for summer camp. Now I have to pay the late fee. I missed the on-time payment for high-school re-application ... late fee again. I accidentally skipped payment on the late notice for the EZ Pass toll; I'm sure to rack up yet another ticket. What day is it? Shit on a stick! It's April 14th and we haven't filed our taxes, or talked about filing them, or even contacted our accountant. What was his name again and where is his email address? I forgot to call my mom for the umpteenth time and now it's too late and she'll be too tired and not lucid enough to talk. Did the dentist already fill the cavity she found at Juliette's last visit six weeks ago or was there a second one? Was I supposed to schedule that? How is the drain output on the neck abscess patient I operated on this morning? When should Milla be evaluated for her braces? When are Scarlett's braces supposed to come off?

I drive home in a daze of endless cataloguing. Then comes the inevitable guilt.

Remember Evelyn.

These are solvable problems … I am not standing at my daughter's bedside, praying her brain will function again. The words "infectious complications," "sepsis," "stroke," "meningitis," and "unknown future" are not whirling around in my precious child's medical chart.

Keep perspective.

I straighten up in the driver's seat, clear my head, and focus on the road.

Tonight, I will choose one undone task to complete at home. Just one. I will not overwhelm myself with the comprehensive list. I will enter my home and remove my shoes. I will not walk around with my coat zipped up and my sneakers still on for two hours because I never took the time to untie them. I will greet my family and absorb the animated chatter about the details of their day. I will not immediately escape into the dark quiet of my bedroom, lie down for "just a second," and fall fast asleep at 8:00 p.m. (only to be awake the rest of the night). I will listen to Alex for at least 10 minutes without immediate interruption by text or email. I will not let my mind drift, belabor, or ruminate over the mistakes I made (or almost made) that day. I will pause and sit cross-legged on the area rug, pet my overly affectionate dogs, and toss their ball. I will kiss and hug whoever lets me, human or fur baby.

I will savor the clamor for attention, cherish the welcoming love, and temper my tendency toward impatience. I will not torture myself with the unintended interpersonal missteps of my day. I will eat only after chewing without shoveling and while actually sitting on a chair. I will make myself tea and, rather than immediately becoming distracted and leaving the teabag to steep endlessly and tea to grow cold, I will drink it.

I will pause before I dive into the deep abyss of others' needs and the mound of personal obligations.

I will inhale and exhale for two whole minutes. I will breathe.

CHAPTER 17

THE TIES THAT BIND

With Gratitude for Nurses

SOME METAL SURGICAL instruments emerging from sterilization can be scorching — often exceeding 200°F (93°C). This intense heat is a byproduct of the sterilization process, which involves either steam (i.e., moist heat at 250-270°F / 121-134°C) or dry heat (320-374°F / 160-190°C). The freshly sterilized instruments must cool before being handled — or you'll burn your hands.

Contrary to popular belief, the biggest rate-limiting step to starting surgery usually isn't the surgeon's availability. It's the system … a vast, intricate network of living and mechanical moving parts. Some days, everything grinds to a halt because we're waiting for clean, cooled instruments. Other days, it's the lack of physical operating room space, or it's the missing Coblator box — with the correct foot pedal. Monitors need proper brightness settings. Navigation systems must be correctly calibrated. There are a hundred small, technical, often finicky details — many tailored to the surgeon's preferences.

And the glue that holds it all together? The nursing staff.

By "nursing staff," I don't just mean those with "RN" after their names. I'm talking about everyone who cares for the patient — scrub techs, anesthesia techs, pre-op and PACU nurses, patient care techs, transporters, and room and instrument cleaners. The ones who fuel the engine that keeps the OR humming.

Yes, the job matters. OR time is expensive. Kids are hungry. Parents are anxious. But what matters most are the people who go above and beyond. Those who anticipate. Those who stay late even when it's tough. Those who give of themselves — often to support us (needy) doctors — even when they feel overlooked or undervalued.

After fifteen years, my morning walk from the locker room to the OR board feels like a stroll through my hometown — natural, comforting, and full of familiar faces.

After fifteen years, my morning walk from the locker room to the OR board feels like a stroll through my hometown — natural, comforting, and full of familiar faces.

"Hey Doc, love your sick new kicks."

I smile.

"Doc, I'm gonna wheel over the microscope from the procedure room as soon as you're done."

Perfect.

"Dr. Lando, I brought up an extra pediatric head and neck tray for your last two cases… in the event something's missing."

Good thinking. Leon, you rock.

"Careful, floor's wet. Just mopped."

Eyes down, skimming patient updates from the team "group chat"
—I almost slip.

"Thanks. Wouldn't want to kick off this hell of a day by landing flat on my ass."

That gets him chuckling.

"Good morning, beautiful!"

Oh, Julio (our anesthesia tech), you say that to everyone … but I blush anyway.

"Tali, have you eaten? I assume not."

Of course not. But thank you for thinking of me.

Ann — the only one who consistently checks in on my nutrition. We met while co-volunteering to register hospital staff for COVID vaccines at the height of the pandemic. She doesn't just leave me her last vanilla protein shake in the lounge — she goes to Panera to get me a cup, straw, and ice to pour it over.

"Doctor Lando! You are so funny."

Jennie — the only nurse I know who willingly left the relative calm of an outpatient surgical center to dive back into the belly of the beast at a tertiary medical center — and once the shock wore off, actually stayed … happily. She's also the only one in the OR lounge who reliably laughs at all my silly anecdotes. (Which makes her basically irreplaceable.)

"Doctor Lando. You need to check out this website with the coolest Star of David jewelry!"

I will.

There's Allison — or Ali — always upbeat, steady, and ready to help, even in the hardest rooms with the trickiest personalities (names withheld to protect the guilty).

There's Christine: no-nonsense, detail-oriented (dare I say sassy), and the only woman in the OR capable of achieving a flawless eyeliner wing-tip.

"How are you doing today, Doctor Lando?"

"I'm good, how are you?"

If it's Gaby asking, the answer is always "great!" She's a genuine ray of sunshine in our insane pressure cooker.

There are several "Michelles" — two in particular, with wildly different personalities and differently spelled names, but both fierce in their commitment to patient safety.

There are the newbies — young nurses and techs, just graduated and thrown into the deep-end. Some sink and leave, but others, like Alexis and Caitlin, float to the top to become the next generation of OR team superstars.

There's the early staff that start us off and the late nurses, like Daisy, who "burn the midnight oil."

There's our "muscle," like Roy — patient care technicians who run around helping, forever moving equipment and transferring patients from OR table to stretcher. In the evenings, there's Charles, the only person in the hospital who calls me simply "Lando," as a term of endearment rather than disrespect (at least I hope).

Of course, there are so many others, too many to capture in these mere pages, those who may not be frequent fliers in my room, but make the daily world go 'round for other surgeons.

"We're opening a second room so you can bounce."

Efficiency. Like music to my ears.

Then there's the OR front desk: Orlando, who would fly around the Earth backward like Superman to make it happen. Lamont — steady, smiling, and generous enough to let me steal his iPhone charger without ever calling me out (or unplugging my phone when I'm not looking).

There are those who constantly help with everything and anything that's not in their job description — like Ilin, the front desk clerk.

And those who keep the whole machine running — Laurie F., Maureen, and Kim C. — and on the backend in the OR scheduling office, Jennifer Little and her crew. Yes, they scold me (frequently) for my unsanctioned zip-up hoodie over scrubs — but they also coordinate the impossible: syncing surgeons, anesthesiologists, pre-op and post-op teams; managing room availability; and somehow still fighting to preserve breaks, lunches, and sanity. They triage the chaos of the add-on list, balancing clinical urgency with staffing reality. And just when every puzzle piece finally fits — bam — an emergency case blows it all up again.

Just when every puzzle piece finally fits — bam — an emergency case blows it all up again.

There's pre-op — sweet, wonderful nurses who settle in and process my patients and comfort anxious kids and their parents, who are even more anxious.

"Doctor Lando, your daughters are so beautiful."

Aww … heart melts. I think so too.

"Doctor Lando, does the 3-month-old airway case need the pediatric ICU post-op?"

"Yes, thanks for checking, Mary."

Crap! I forgot to call them.

"Don't worry, I'll call them."

Later ...

"Did you remember to mark the patient?"

No, I will now.

"Did you remember to sign the H&P?"

No again, I will now.

There's post-op — the nurses who monitor, stabilize, and comfort young patients as they transition from anesthetic sleep to wakefulness. They handle post-op pain and nausea, and weather the turbulence of emergence delirium. They reassure our patients' parents about what's normal and educate them about what's not.

Back in the OR ...

"Hi, Tali. How was your weekend?"

"Frannie!!! If you ever fully retire, I'll have to quit my job."

"Tali, you'll be fine without me."

"No. Actually I won't!"

Ok ... time to get this party started. Let me find chilaxing music. Mumford and Sons, Lumineers, and U2.

Time out. I need a ...

"Here you go."

David hands me the instrument that I need before I can even formulate its name.

Thank you.

"How are your girls? Show me Juliette's newest artwork? She's mad talented."

~~~

Later …

"Hey Maureen, who's gonna stay late and cover my room for the late add-on cases?"

"Hannah offered to stay for you … again."

Of course she did. Love her!

It's been said that I'm impatient, entitled, overly particular — even brusque. Some might go so far as to call me bitchy.

I know. I know. I'll try not to be.

I've been told I tend to rush people, push too hard to get the cases going.

I do. But please understand — it's not for me.

I've been reminded (many, many times) to sign my notes, finish my charts, and submit my damn resident evaluations and time-study reports.

I get so busy. I meant to.

Loud roar. It's a Tiger Text. Marked priority. From Minimol Mathia:

> DR. LANDO — I'M BEGGING YOU. PLEASE COMPLETE YOUR OP NOTE!

~~~

This is my love letter and my thank you to "my crew" — to those dedicated, wonderful individuals who forgive my sins and grant me grace for my vast imperfections. To those who show me kindness even when I'm rough around the edges. To those members of the nursing staff who make me look good, make it all happen — all day, every day — for our deserving patients and make time and space for the unexpected.

This is my acknowledgment that we are only as successful as the team that lifts us up. The patient and their families don't get to meet all the people who helped or saved their child. But, from the inside, I see them clearly.

CHAPTER 18

MY BREAD AND BUTTER

BEYOND THE RIVETING stories shared here, much of my time follows a more formulaic pattern: I spend three days a week in the clinic — Tuesdays, Wednesdays, and Fridays — and the other two days in the operating room. Most pediatric ENT issues I manage in the outpatient setting involve hearing problems, ear infections, nasal congestion, and snoring. My special areas of interest are swallowing dysfunction and noisy-breathing infants. The most common ambulatory surgical procedures I perform include adenotonsillectomy, ear tube placement, control of nosebleeds, and inferior turbinate reductions.

The patient populations I care for are widely diverse. Although my practice is based in an affluent area, the demographics of my patients are far from what you might expect. I have satellite offices across the bridge and far up north. At least half of my patients come from underserved communities. Many don't speak English, so my medical Spanglish is pretty good — though we always use professional interpreters.

My favorite — and sizable — subset of patients comes from the foster care system. Their backstories are often shocking. Many start life at a tremendous disadvantage, exposed in utero to polysub-stance use and frequently victims of neglect or abuse. As a result, many face neurological impairments, developmental delays, and autism spectrum disorders.

I'm consistently in awe of the fortitude of their foster parents — whether biological relatives or not. Though their stories are gut-wrenching, I feel honored to be part of their care. Helping them to hear better, to breathe more easily, or to improve feeding gives me profound purpose.

Despite the routine nature of their problems and interventions, this work is deeply fulfilling. I watch these children grow, seeing the lucky ones thrive while many still struggle mightily long-term. Even when the work is monotonous, the intensity of their need fuels and recharges me.

Though I often feel harried, I truly enjoy teaching. Many of my clinic and OR days include at least one medical student, physician assistant student, or resident shadowing me. Part of my academic duties also involves giving lectures on topics like "Pediatric Obstruc-tive Sleep Apnea," "Infant Noisy Breathing," "Pediatric Swallowing Disorders" (related to ENT), and "Endoscopic Airway Surgery."

I savor the rush of public speaking. Having delivered numerous professional talks in otolaryngology and author-related presenta-tions for my first book, *Hell & Back*, I've often been told I'm an engaging lecturer. Though I haven't yet given a network television interview, I aspire to — perhaps this book will open that door.

All in all, I have the best of both worlds. Most of my days are relatively predictable, but the smattering of stimulating and unusual cases is enough to keep me on my toes. I'm constantly busy but do have autonomous control of my schedule (which is not always the case these days in medicine). I have colleagues and support staff (like a wonderful office PA named Melis) — seasoned and new — who I like and respect. I have senior colleagues like Dr. Augustine Muscatello, who has bestowed to me decades of advice, and Dr. David Merer, who graciously covers my call when I'm in a bind. At the midpoint of my career, I am still learning and growing and acquiring new skills. Admittedly, I am perceived as demanding and often over-stretched and over-stressed. But I have a team of dedicated people around me, including my office managers — past and present (Vivian, Christina, Donnie, and Liz) — and my "work-wives," including my long-standing and infinitely trustworthy medical assistants (Christine R. and others). Angelica V., my surgery-scheduler extraordinaire, not only masterminds my OR schedule but also buys me a yogurt parfait for breakfast because she knows I'd otherwise go all day without eating. Britney R. spoils me on Tuesdays with Dunkin Donuts two-shot coconut coffees with two Splendas or a venti chai with soy milk from Starbucks. There are also a dizzying array of front desk, scheduling, and answering-service personnel without whom my whole world would not turn.

At the midpoint of my career, I am still learning and growing and acquiring new skills.

So, despite the constant threat of burnout, the overwhelming headaches of modern medicine's challenges and charting systems, the ubiquitous dysfunction of the hospital, and the relentless staff turnover — despite all the phone calls, late nights, and early mornings — I know one thing for sure… I still love what I do.

CHAPTER 19

IT'S GONNA TAKE
YOUR BREATH AWAY

IN ANY JOB — even the most inherently fulfilling ones — you need to figure out what fuels your fire. Medicine is no different. For me, in addition to caring for children, it is the solving of complex enigmas, the collaboration with people who I admire, and, yes, it's the high stakes too. As a surgeon, you need to accept that in the operating room, the buck will always stop with you. No matter what. Some days, you will feel triumphant. Many days, you will feel like Atlas bearing the weight of the world on your shoulders. On the very worst days, you will be Icarus free-falling from the sky.

As a surgeon, you need to accept that in the operating room, the buck will always stop with you. No matter what. Some days, you will feel triumphant. Many days, you will feel like Atlas bearing the weight of the world on your shoulders. On the very worst days, you will be Icarus free-falling from the sky.

Considering all this, I can offer some advice to those who are reading this book during their undergraduate pre-med journey: Think hard before you choose this profession. It's a long, long haul. Be sure it is all you ever wanted or, at the very least, what you think you want. Next, arm yourself with grit, reliance, endurance, and dedication. Be honest with yourself. Ask yourself, "Do I possess these qualities?" Make sure the answer is "yes." You will need them.

Then, construct an evolving phalanx of trusted colleagues, mentors, friends, and family. You will indisputably lean on them. Find your "sounding boards" — those people you can bounce ideas off and who will listen when things get tough. The members of your support structure may change depending on the situation. For me, there are many.

Aside from my husband and rock (Alex) and highly-competent practice partners (many of whom I've already mentioned), there is also Steve Hemmerdinger (my Tuesday and Wednesday office-buddy and confidant) and Dave Garber (our laryngologist and my pediatric voice clinic collaborator and co-surgeon). There are my siblings (Zvi, Dov and J.J.) and my extraordinary (and very tolerant of my shortcomings) sisters-in-law (Betty and Debra). There is also Dr. Mike Rutter, my yoda, Dr. Eli Grunstein, my moral compass, and a more extended network of core med school and residency friends (Avital, Natalie, Miki, and Caroline, to name a few) and countless wonderful physicians (available by immediate text) from pediatrics and other subspecialties, such as Pulmonology, Infectious Disease, GI, Allergy/Immunology, and Hematology/Oncology. Beyond professional ties, I still rely on my deepest friendships, like Avigail B., and my tight circle of local friends, such as the "Lovely Ladies of White Plains," and other saviors (you know who you are) for emergency picking up of my kids, feeding my dogs, maintaining my sanity, and enabling me to sleep at night … at least some of the time.

Future surgeons: Once you've decided this life is for you and once you've begun gathering allies to see you through, strap yourself in for the bumpy road ahead. It will be hard — at times all-consuming and demanding — but it will also be spectacular and exhilarating. No matter what you expect, it's gonna take your breath away.

EPILOGUE

The Deepest Dive

THE ONLY RECREATIONAL sport I have ever loved is scuba diving. The first time I sank beneath the ocean's surface was the first time I ever felt truly still. There was no noise except the low-frequency ambient sounds of gas bubbles and my steady breath through the regulator … in and out. There were no surrounding distractions. There were just the dazzling colors of the tropical fish and the vibrant coral. One exhilarating experience and I was hooked. Until that point, I had only a singular focus of my entire adult life — to become a doctor. In scuba diving, I finally found a physical, non-academic passion too.

It took me 15 more years to find true love. I fell for Alex the moment I heard his voice. Before we even met — though yes, I had seen his hot picture — I knew he was the one. Maybe it was because I was already in my 30s, navigating the brutally competitive New York City Jewish singles scene. Maybe it was because I'd kissed more than my share of frogs. Hell, I'd even married — and divorced — one. Whatever the case may be, I knew from our very first conversation that this was a person who understood me. This was a man who I could be completely myself around. I didn't have to hide my obsessive perfectionism or my punishing insecurities. I didn't have to bury my neurotic stress — though I'm sure there are times he wishes I would. Most importantly, he was someone who always built me up, never tore me down. Over the years, he hasn't just forgiven my countless mistakes, broken plans, or forgotten promises — he's always accepted them as part of the deal.

I knew from our very first conversation that this was a person who understood me. This was a man who I could be completely myself around.

Alex proposed to me beneath the clear waters of Bonaire. The diamond ring was wrapped around his neck with twine, and he dangled it in front of me until I nodded my head "yes." The funny thing about it all was that he hated the experience of scuba diving. But he knew it was special to me and so he gallantly persevered. As soon as I agreed to marry him, he shot up from the depths immediately and has never been back down.

The raw truth about being married to a surgeon is that it's not pretty. Despite the fulfillment, it's an all-encompassing, sometimes punishing, and thoroughly taxing job. By night, I really need to decompress. Alex and I spend a lot of time together just being in the same place, watching TV, being quiet (not always a joint decision). We rewatch our beloved shows like *Modern Family* and *Veep* because they are funny, mindless, and calming. I need that and he knows it.

As ridiculous and mortifying as our children find it, we thoroughly enjoy quoting our favorite lines and laughing uncontrollably.

Alex is an exquisite amateur chef. When I truly crave comfort, he makes me this Vietnamese soup made with broth, rice noodles, meat, and herbs called Pho.

"Is it Phah or Pho?" (From the *Modern Family* episode "Run for Your Life," in which Mitch and Cam tell their Asian doctor that they plan on raising Lily in her Asian heritage. Cameron asks if he pronounced the name of an Asian soup correctly, but Dr. Miura is from Denver — not Asia — and takes offense to it.)

Offering me these delicious dishes is a true act of love, and his startling grasp of the umami flavor is nothing short of a culinary triumph. More than that, it's just one more way he intuitively gives me the kind of support I need, exactly when I need it.

Don't misunderstand, though — managing work, family, and relationships is a delicate affair. After more than a decade and a half of trying to decipher the "special sauce," Alex and I have been through many iterations of "us" with effort, failure, and recalibration. When we were both working full-time and the kids were babies, we had live-in nannies. It was a rollercoaster — there were wonderful, loving, lifelong connections, but also many points of crisis. This wasn't a luxury; it was an expensive necessity. We had no nearby grandparents or relatives to consistently lean on (although my in-laws, Mark and Anna, have saved us many times from childcare failure). All our friends were also working full-time, facing the same realities of raising families.

After many years, we transitioned to an au pair model. It worked well for shuttling the kids and basic meal prep, but frequent turnover, visa issues, and unexpected car damage made it challenging. In recent years, as our girls have become teens and preteens, their needs have grown more complex — and demand more parental involvement. Unfortunately, this has coincided with a significant increase in my professional workload. As a result, Alex has taken on many of the core responsibilities of psychological, medical, and dental care in addition to carpooling and tutor shuttling.

Though there are precious moments of perfect bliss, our family life is a constant work in progress. We feel our way forward through trial and error — mostly error — and shared decision-making. We bicker (though I wish we didn't), argue (to our kids' chagrin), and demonstrate our individual flaws more often than we'd like. We're wildly different people yet surprisingly aligned in our core values. Because of that, we usually agree on the big decisions, but often struggle with execution and the daily details. All I know for certain is that we love the world we've built together — the beautiful children we've raised, our dogs (some might say too much), our home, and our community of family and friends. Despite the ongoing challenge of achieving the right balance, it's an ideal worth fighting for.

After my bilateral mastectomies and lymph node dissection for locally metastatic breast cancer, I was told I should never scuba dive again. The main risk after a complete axillary node dissection is developing lymphedema in the affected arm due to pressure changes underwater. Lymphedema occurs when lymph fluid builds up in tissues because the lymphatic system — responsible for draining excess fluid — has been disrupted by surgery. Symptoms include a feeling of fullness, heaviness, or tightness in the arm, itching, burning, and significant swelling. These changes can be reversible or permanent. There's no cure for lymphadema, but it can be managed through exercise, wrapping, compression, and specialized physical therapy. It's also not a great aesthetic — having one "elephant arm," especially for a surgeon who wears short-sleeved scrubs. Even now, at baseline, years after surgery, my left arm remains visibly larger than my right.

Of all the consequences of having breast cancer at a young age — and the treatments that followed, which included, to name just a few, inability to have more children (which I wanted), body image struggles, fear of mortality, emotional turmoil, and an increased risk of cardio-vascular disease — the "no scuba-diving" restriction hit me especially hard. For years, I followed the rules. But in the end, we all make choices that balance what serves our bodies with what feeds our souls.

The first time I returned to the watery depths, I feared the conse-quences. Instead of diving into the warm Caribbean Sea, I opted for a shallow dive off a small pier along the cold waters of the Saint Lawrence River near the Thousand Islands at the US-Canadian border. As I swam along the bow of the steel cargo steamer SS Keystorm's shipwreck, I was awestruck by its massive forward wheelhouse. Then, I angled down to the riverbed where I hovered, buoyant, watching a smallmouth bass glide by. The sound of the rushing water filled my senses, drowning out the competing voices in my head. After months of living at a frenetic pace without respite, I finally found some peace. And when I emerged back on the surface, I could breathe again.

CHASING DREAMS

ON A FAMILY trip to Greece a year and a half ago, while my children played with their cousins, I found a quiet moment alone in my hotel room and opened my laptop to begin this book. The first stories poured out — years of experiences, memories, and patients I'd carried in my mind and heart, finally released. But after that cathartic outpouring, I hit a wall. Breathless was my dream — but how would I find the time to write it? And even if I did, would anyone care?

The answer to the first question is twofold. Writing has always brought me immense satisfaction and joy, so I made the time. I squeezed it into every little crack of my day. I began carrying my laptop everywhere. Instead of pacing outside the OR during turnover, I wrote. During the 90-minute drive to my satellite office up north, I dictated voice memos into my phone. While my daughters did homework at the kitchen table, I sat beside them, furiously typing. While they skied (I do not), I babysat the dogs in the lodge, absorbed in the creative process. Somehow, time seemed to stretch to fit this passion project. But time is a precious, limited commodity — you have to beg, borrow, and steal it. And so I did.

Kate Colbert, who became my editor and publisher, answered the second question for me. When I first reached out for help, she wasn't taking new clients. She offered to be an ad hoc writing coach but couldn't commit to the full process. Then, six months later, seemingly out of the blue, Kate reached out. She told me she'd thought of me, bought my first book, *Hell & Back*, and taken it poolside on a trip. Once she started reading, she couldn't put it down.

"I love your writing. I want to work with you. I'll make the time. Please send me the manuscript for the new book."

It's hard to describe the surge of adrenaline her faith gave me. Someone believed in me — someone discerning, with vast experience — a writer, editor, and publisher. Not my ever-approving mother, nor my supportive husband — an outsider with no skin in the game.

That was the turning point. From then on, we were in this together. **I was all in.**

ACKNOWLEDGMENTS

THERE ARE SO many people to thank — people without whom this book would not have been possible.

To my early readers and cheerleaders: **Rhonda Rose, Fran Salzano,** and my daughters **Scarlett and Juliette**.

To my generous endorsers: **Dr. Samuel Barst, Kristin Bernstein, Dr. Linda Bluestein, Lizbeth Meredith**, **Dr. Chris Park, Dr. Alok Patel,** and **Dr. Sue Varma**.

Thank you **to the editor at Random House who rejected my first book** — even though she said she "loved my voice" — but encouraged me to "get back to me when you write another book about a female surgeon who loves to scuba dive." I didn't get back to her, but I did write that book. You're holding it in your hands.

Thank you again to **Kate Colbert**, my writing coach, editor, and publisher, for truly believing in me, encouraging me, and helping turn this wonderful dream into a tightly written reality. Kate, the more I know you, the more I am impressed with the vastness of your experience, the depth of your knowledge, and your dedication to your authors. You are filled with invaluable ideas and insights. What started as a professional relationship has blossomed into a deep mutual respect. Despite your personal medical struggles, you never fail to answer my texts, jump on calls, and guide me through this process with love, enthusiasm, and brilliance.

Thanks also to the rest of the Silver Tree Publishing team, especially to **George Stevens**, who took my vague idea and transformed it into the most gorgeous and powerful cover. I am so lucky you are part of my winning team.

Thank you to my publicist, **Emily Florence**, for championing me and for believing in the power of this book to touch hearts and change lives. Whereas everyone else told me, "success will be a steep, vertical climb," Emily said, "tell me your dreams and I'll make them happen." We were an immediate "dream team!"

Thank you to my next-door neighbor and friend, **Louis Goldstein**, who painstakingly combed through the finished manuscript, offering valuable insights, intelligent modifications, and grammatical fine-tuning (which he feared were nitpicky but I found were superbly elevating).

Thank you to my resident, **Dr. Maria Mavrommatis**, who generously sacrificed her limited personal time to read and offer invaluable insights on my rough drafts.

Thank you to **all my superstar residents** who tolerate my repetition, appreciate my sarcasm, and forgive me my neurotic behavior when it comes to pediatric patients. Collectively and individually, you have stood in the trenches with me, pushed me to be a lifelong learner, and taught me as much as I have taught you.

Thank you again **to all the amazing colleagues** I mentioned in the "My Bread and Butter" chapter.

Thank you again to **Dr. Mike Rutter**. Aside from writing a phenomenal and touching foreword, he has been a faithful early reader of all my chapters and advisor for all things, big and small.

Thank you **to my mother, Susan Lando**, for always believing in me, especially in my creative writing, even since I was a young girl. Thank you for the countless hours you spent with me reading chapters out loud, listening to the cadence of the sentences, and then painstakingly revising the grammar and word choices. Your gradual memory loss has been a devastating reality for you and the many of us who love you. Working with you on this book has been my most treasured opportunity to highlight that your intelligence and wisdom remains intact despite the cruel ravages of cognitive decline.

And most importantly, **to my phenomenally supportive husband Alex** and **to my gorgeous — inside and out — daughters, Juliette, Scarlett, and Milla.** You are all the answers to the frequently asked question, "How the hell did you have time to write another book?" Thank you for enabling and encouraging me to continue following my dreams. Thank you for the million ways you allow me to be a wife, mother, doctor, and author.

GLOSSARY OF TERMS
AND ABBREVIATIONS

THROUGHOUT THE STORIES in *Breathless* are many medical terms and abbreviations. While we have endeavored to define and explain these terms and acronyms in the contexts in which they are introduced, we know it can be additionally helpful to have a go-to Glossary for easy-to-understand explanations and clarifications. We hope this special section of the book helps non-medical readers follow the surgical stories and understand the procedures, conditions, and tools referenced throughout.

COMMON ABBREVIATIONS

ADHD   Attention-Deficit/Hyperactivity Disorder

ALTE   Apparent Life-Threatening Event

COVID Coronavirus Disease (the condition caused by the SARS-CoV2 virus)

CPAP   Continuous Positive Airway Pressure

CPR   Cardiopulmonary Resuscitation

CT   Computed Tomography (scan)

EKG   Electrocardiogram

ENT	Ear, Nose, and Throat (physician specialty, more formally known as otolaryngology)
EMT	Emergency Medical Technician
ER	Emergency Room (also **ED** Emergency Department)
EXIT	Ex Utero Intrapartum Treatment
GA	General Anesthesia
H&P	History and Physical (examination)
ICU	Intensive Care Unit
IV	Intravenous
MRI	Magnetic Resonance Imaging
NG	Nasogastric (tube)
NICU	Neonatal Intensive Care Unit
NPO	*Nil Per Os* (nothing by mouth)
OR	Operating Room
PALS	Pediatric Advanced Life Support
PICU	Pediatric Intensive Care Unit
PPE	Personal Protective Equipment
T&A	Tonsillectomy and Adenoidectomy

GLOSSARY OF TERMS

15-Blade Scalpel

A small, curved blade with a sharp, rounded tip used especially for delicate incisions in pediatric surgery.

Abscess

A localized collection of pus that forms within tissue due to infection.

Acute Sphenoid Sinusitis

Sudden-onset infection of the sphenoid sinus, one of the four pairs of paranasal sinuses located deep in the skull, behind the nasal cavity and between the eyes.

Adenoidectomy

An adenoidectomy is the surgical removal of the adenoids, tissue located at the back of the nasal cavity.

Adenotonsillectomy

An adenotonsillectomy removes both the adenoids and tonsils, often to improve breathing or prevent recurrent infections.

Admission

The formal process of being accepted into a hospital for care, usually because a patient needs treatment, monitoring, or surgery that cannot be done safely as an outpatient.

Airway

The airway is the passage that carries air from the nose and mouth to the lungs.

Anesthesia

Anesthesia is medication that prevents pain and keeps a patient unconscious or sedated during surgery.

Anesthesiologist

An anesthesiologist is a doctor who administers anesthesia and monitors patients during surgery.

Apparent Life-Threatening Event (ALTE)

An ALTE is when an infant suddenly stops breathing or changes color but is later revived.

Attending

A fully trained, board-certified doctor who has completed all residency and fellowship training. Attending surgeons hold ultimate responsibility for patient care, perform or supervise operations, and make final medical decisions.

Aspiration

Aspiration means inhaling food, liquid, or foreign objects into the airway or lungs instead of swallowing into the esophagus.

Bair Hugger

A Bair Hugger is a warming device used during surgery to maintain a patient's body temperature.

Biopsy

A biopsy is the removal of a small tissue sample for examination under a microscope.

Bouffant

In medicine, it is a type of disposable hair covering worn in sterile environments like operating rooms. It's shaped like a puff or balloon to accommodate various hair volumes.

Breaking Scrub

Breaking scrub is when a surgeon or nurse or assistant leaves the sterile field and cannot return without hand/arm washing, replacing their gown, and putting on new sterile gloves.

Bronchopulmonary Dysplasia

Bronchopulmonary dysplasia is a chronic lung disease often seen in premature infants who required long-term ventilation.

Bronchoscope / Rigid Bronchoscope

A metal tube of various sizes with a camera used to view the airway and lungs.

Bronchoscopy

A bronchoscopy is a procedure using a bronchoscope to examine or treat problems in the airway or lungs. Performed for both diagnosis and foreign-body removal.

Cannula (Nasal Cannula)

A small plastic tube with prongs that are inserted in the nostrils used for delivering supplemental oxygen (or sometimes other medical gases).

Cerebritis

Inflammation of the brain tissue (the cerebrum). It is typically an early stage of a brain infection and may precede the formation of a brain abscess.

Combustible

Refers to materials or gases that can easily ignite or burn in the operating room, especially during airway procedures where oxygen levels are high. Electrocautery ("Bovie") and lasers used in airway surgery increase the risk of combustion.

Continuous Positive Airway Pressure (CPAP)

CPAP is a type of air delivery system that delivers constant air pressure to keep the airway open using a plastic face mask or nasal prongs.

Crepitus

Crackling, popping, or grating sensation or sound that can be felt or heard under the skin, in joints, or in soft tissues caused by air trapped under the skin.

Debrief

A debrief is a post-surgery discussion about what went well and what could be improved. Debriefs are intended to improve outcomes and teamwork.

Decannulate

The process of permanently removing a tracheostomy tube when it is no longer needed for breathing or airway support.

Dura

The outermost, thickest, and toughest layer of the protective coverings (called meninges) that surround the brain and spinal cord.

Electrocautery

A common surgical tool that uses electric current to cut tissue or stop bleeding.

Embolus (Emboli, plural)

A clot that breaks loose and travels through the blood until it lodges in a vessel that's too small for it to pass, causing a sudden blockage.

Endotracheal Tube

An endotracheal tube is a breathing tube inserted into the windpipe during intubation.

Endoscopic Surgery

Endoscopic surgery uses small cameras and instruments inserted through natural or openings such as the nose or mouth to perform procedures. Endoscopic airway procedures address common airway problems in infants and children.

Epistaxis

Epistaxis is the medical term for a nosebleed.

EXIT Procedure

The EXIT procedure is a surgery performed while a baby remains connected to the umbilical cord in order to provide continued oxygen from the mother's blood while the airway is secured.

Extubation

The process of taking out a previously placed breathing tube from the trachea (windpipe) once the patient can breathe on their own.

Fistula

A fistula is an abnormal connection between two epithelialized surfaces (meaning two areas lined with cells like skin or mucous membrane) that are not normally connected.

In the case of a tracheocutaneous fistula, it is a persistent tract between the trachea (windpipe) and the skin of the neck.

Foreign Body Aspiration

Foreign body aspiration occurs when an object is inhaled and becomes lodged in the airway or lungs.

Granulation Tissue

Granulation tissue is the new, healing tissue that forms during the repair of a wound. It is a normal part of wound healing and filling in defects from injury but often becomes excessive, thereby causing problems.

Hemostasis

The process of stopping bleeding through medical techniques, such as pressure, sutures, electrocautery, or medications. Achieving hemostasis is a critical step in surgery to maintain a clear field and major prevent blood loss.

Hypothermia

Hypothermia is a dangerous drop in body temperature, which can be during surgery by using warming devices like the Bair Hugger.

Intubation

Intubation is the placement of a breathing tube into the windpipe to maintain an open airway.

Larynx

The larynx, or voice box, sits in the throat and helps produce sound and protect the airway. This structure is often examined during airway surgeries.

Laryngoscope

A laryngoscope is a tool used to view the larynx and insert breathing tubes and is used in nearly all airway procedures.

Laryngospasm

Laryngospasm is when the vocal cords suddenly clamp shut, blocking airflow.

Laser Surgery

Laser surgery uses focused light beams to cut or vaporize tissue.

Level-1 Trauma

Level 1 trauma centers are referral hubs for smaller hospitals (Level 2–4). They not only treat the most critically injured patients but also serve as leaders in trauma system organization, teaching, and innovation.

Lymph Node

A lymph node is a small, bean-shaped structure located in multiple clusters in various areas in the body. It is part of the lymphatic system, which plays a key role in your body's immune defense.

Microlaryngeal Instruments

Microlaryngeal instruments are fine tools used for delicate surgeries on the vocal cords or airway.

Morbidity

Refers to the medical complications associated with a procedure for an individual.

Nasogastric (NG) Tube

A nasogastric tube (often abbreviated NG tube) is a flexible, hollow tube that's inserted through the nose, down the esophagus, and into the stomach, used to deliver food and medications.

Nasopharynx

The nasopharynx is the uppermost part of the throat (pharynx), located behind the nose and above the soft palate. The nasopharynx is the transition zone between the nose and the throat.

Neonatal Intensive Care Unit (NICU)

The NICU is a hospital unit that cares for critically ill or premature newborns.

Nidus

The source, such as a source of infection.

Otolaryngologist

An otolaryngologist is a doctor who specializes in treating the ear, nose, and throat (ENT).

Pediatric Intensive Care Unit (PICU)

The PICU provides intensive care for critically ill children.

Phlegmon

A diffuse infection within soft tissue, often causing inflammation, swelling, and pain. Unlike an abscess, a phlegmon is more ill-defined and is often treated with IV antibiotics instead of surgical drainage.

Posterior

The back wall of the trachea or windpipe.

Purulence

Purulence means the presence or production of pus. Purulence is a sign of infection, typically bacterial, because pus forms as the immune system fights invading microbes

Preemie (and Micro-Preemie)

Preemie and micro-preemie are informal terms used to describe babies born prematurely — meaning before the standard 37 weeks of pregnancy. The difference is in *how early* they are born. A micro-preemie is a baby born extremely early, usually before 26-28 weeks gestation and/or weighing less than 1,000 grams (about 2.2 pounds).

Pulmonary Edema

Pulmonary edema is fluid buildup in the lungs that makes breathing difficult.

Resident

A physician-in-training who has graduated from medical school and is now undergoing specialized training in a particular field of medicine.

Retropharyngeal Abscess

A retropharyngeal abscess is a collection of pus in the retropharyngeal space — the area behind the pharynx (throat) and in front of the cervical spine.

Rigid bronchoscopy

Rigid bronchoscopy uses a stiff tube to examine or remove blockages in the airway.

Septic

When a patient is in the state of a life-threatening, body-wide response to infection that can lead to organ dysfunction or failure.

Sphenoid Sinus

One of the four pairs of paranasal sinuses, which are air-filled spaces located deep in the skull behind the nasal cavity between the eyes.

Stenosis

An abnormal narrowing of the airway in the larynx (voice box) or trachea (windpipe), which may result from trauma, prolonged intubation, infection, inflammation, or congenital conditions.

Stoma

A tracheostoma is the surgically created opening in the front of the neck that connects the trachea (windpipe) to the skin surface.

Stridor

A high-pitched, noisy breathing sound that signals a blocked or narrowed airway.

Subglottic Cyst

A fluid-filled growth just below the vocal cords, which can obstruct airflow. It is often   found in premature infants who have had a long periods of intubation in the past.

Suprastomal Stent

A plastic stent used to maintain airway patency (i.e., to keep the airway open) in patients who have undergone airway reconstructive surgery.

Surfactant

Surfactant is a substance in the lungs that keeps the air sacs open. Premature babies often lack surfactant, leading to breathing difficulties.

Surgical Time-Out

A surgical time-out is a ritual pause before surgery to confirm specific patient details and ensure safety.

Tonsillectomy

A tonsillectomy is the surgical reduction or removal of the tonsils, which is often done to treat sleep or infection problems in children.

Tachycardia

A faster-than-normal heart rate.

Thyroidectomy

A surgical procedure to remove all or part of the thyroid gland, an organ that plays a critical role in regulating metabolism, heart rate, and energy through the production of thyroid hormones.

Trachea

The trachea, or windpipe, is the tube that carries air from the throat to the lungs.

Tracheomalacia

Tracheomalacia is when the windpipe walls are weak and collapse, making breathing difficult.

Tracheostomy (or "Trach")

A tracheostomy is the surgery to create an opening in the windpipe to help a person breathe.

Tracheotomy (See *Tracheostomy*)

Turbinate

A curved, bony structure inside the nose that is covered with soft tissue and a mucous membrane covering that helps regulate air flow and helps filter, warm, and humidify the air you breathe through your nose.

ABOUT THE AUTHOR

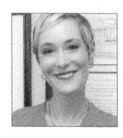 DR. TALI LANDO IS A highly respected board-certified pediatric otolaryngologist and complex airway expert whose rigorous clinical practice and narrative gifts converge in *Breathless: Surgical Tales from the Brink (and Back)*. A summa cum laude graduate in Neuroscience from Columbia University, she earned her MD with honors from Weill Cornell Medical College. An 11-year post-graduate training path followed: a general surgery internship, a five-year Otolaryngology–Head and Neck Surgery residency at New York–Presbyterian Hospital, and fellowship training in pediatric otolaryngology and airway surgery at the Children's Hospital of Philadelphia. She is boarded in Complex Pediatric Otolaryngology.

Dr. Lando serves on the faculty at Westchester Medical Health Network and is an attending pediatric ENT surgeon at Maria Fareri Children's Hospital. Her surgical expertise spans advanced pediatric airway reconstruction, tracheostomy management, endoscopic and open laryngeal procedures, management of adenotonsillar disease, congenital neck masses, and swallowing and sleep disorders in children. Highly regarded by colleagues, she is known for her precision, multidisciplinary collaboration, and firm leadership during critical cases.

Her academic responsibilities include Assistant Professor of Clinical Otolaryngology at Touro Medical College. She is a member of the American Academy of Otolaryngology–Head & Neck Surgery and the American Society of Pediatric Otolaryngology. Dr. Lando has contributed numerous peer-reviewed publications, book chapters, and presentations in high-impact medical journals and conferences.

As an author, she gained recognition with her first memoir, *Hell & Back: Wife & Mother, Doctor & Patient, Dragon Slayer*, chronicling her physician-patient journey through Stage IIIC breast cancer while balancing surgical practice and motherhood. Dr. Lando has been an invited speaker at medical symposia, literary events, podcasts, and patient-centric forums, bridging clinical insight with personal narrative to illuminate the emotional and ethical dimensions of pediatric airway surgery. In a 2022 feature by *ENT Today*, she was highlighted among notable otolaryngologists-turned-authors — a nod to her storytelling prowess.

Her second book, *Breathless*, offers an unflinching look inside pediatric operating rooms — revealing not just technical mastery, but also the human stakes behind each airway case. Beyond the OR, she supports the next generation of surgeons through teaching, mentoring, and integrating narrative reflection into medical education.

Dr. Lando lives in Westchester County, New York, with her husband and three daughters.

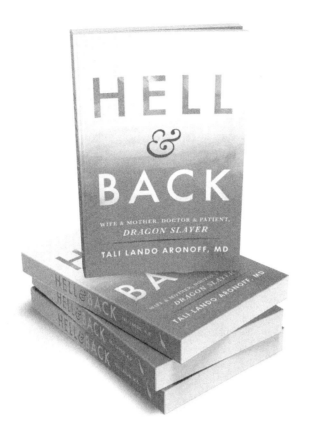

ALSO BY DR. TALI LANDO

If you laughed, cried, or held your breath with *Breathless* ... don't miss where it all began.

Hell & Back: Wife & Mother, Doctor & Patient, Dragon Slayer is Dr. Tali Lando's raw, witty, and unflinching debut memoir about facing breast cancer at the height of her medical career and motherhood. With the same sharp humor and emotional honesty, she brings readers into the trenches of trauma, resilience, and the fight for her life — and back.

Available everywhere books are sold.

GO BEYOND THE BOOK

To learn more about Dr. Lando, to invite her to speak at your event or organization, to order books in bulk, and to connect in meaningful ways, visit **www.DrTaliLando.com.**

Made in United States
North Haven, CT
27 December 2025